Taking Control

Manage stress to get the most out of life

Wayne Froggatt

HarperCollinsPublishers

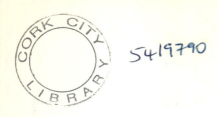

National Library of New Zealand Cataloguing-in-Publication Data

Froggatt, Wayne.
Taking control : manage stress to get the most out of life /
Wayne Froggatt.
ISBN 1-86950-582-4
1. Stress management. 2. Stress (Psychology) 3. Cognitive
therapy. I. Title.
155.9042—dc 22

First published 2006
HarperCollins*Publishers (New Zealand) Limited*
P.O. Box 1, Auckland

ISBN 1 86950 582 4

Cover design by Geeza Design
Cover image courtesy of Getty Images
Internal text typesetting by Island Bridge

Printed by Griffin Press, Australia, on 79 gsm Bulky Paperback

Contents

Acknowledgements

As with my previous books, many of the contributors to *Taking Control* will remain anonymous — the clients who have used the methods described in these pages, and who, over the years, have provided me with feedback which has helped me refine the methods.

I also owe a debt to colleagues who have assisted me with the earlier book *GoodStress*, from which much of the material for *Taking Control* has been developed. I am especially grateful to David Ramsden, Sonya Mason, Julie Parkinson, Dr Paul Hendy, Jenni McKinley, Dr Ruth Williams, Cathi Pharazyn and Greta Wham, who provided me with invaluable guidance, feedback and comments on specific topics relating to their specialist areas of expertise.

This book, like the others, is solidly based on the principles of Cognitive Behaviour Therapy (CBT). Accordingly, I acknowledge an ongoing debt to Drs Albert Ellis and Aaron Beck. To this list, I add two more innovators. First, Dr Dominic DiMattia, the originator of Rational Effectiveness Training, who has developed CBT for use in the workplace (and who kindly provided an introduction to *GoodStress*). Secondly, I am indebted to Professor Stephen Palmer of London, a world authority on cognitive-behavioural approaches to stress management, not only for providing the introduction to *Taking Control*, but also for his contribution to expanding the use of this elegant and effective methodology in New Zealand. I hope that this book will prove to be a worthy addition to the growing literature on rational approaches to personal and workplace effectiveness.

Wayne Froggatt
2006

Introduction

Stress and control: the two are intrinsically linked. If you feel in control of a situation, even a challenging one, you will experience less stress than another person in a similar situation who does not feel in control. This is not rocket science. It is just plain common sense. Modern models of stress, resilience and performance emphasise the importance of empowering people to increase control over their environment to reduce stress and enhance their physical and mental health.

Unfortunately, in many situations — for example, constant change, public speaking, relationships and finance — we may feel out of control. Do you find that you become stressed, angry, anxious or depressed too easily? So often we react with stress to external triggering events, such as a manager's sloppy behaviour or a partner's untidiness. You may wonder: how can I gain control over situations to reduce my stress level?

We may feel like shooting the manager or shouting at our partner, but these are not recommended solutions! Wayne Froggatt, author of *Taking Control*, shows that there are other options to deal with stress and regain control. Most significantly, if we modify how we view stressful events or situations and use the techniques of rational thinking, we can then control how much stress we feel.

Taking Control is full of techniques and strategies to help the reader take control, to reduce their stress and improve their performance. Yes, and perhaps even achieve their life goals. The techniques for modifying thinking and changing behaviours will enhance practical skills such as assertion and time management. All the reader has to do is provide the effort to learn the techniques and then put them into action. Some hard work and practice are needed, but acting on the strategies in *Taking Control* can change lives for the better.

Taking Control can be considered as a self-coaching handbook without having to see a coach. I don't need to wish you good luck if you want to take control. All you have to do is read this book and start using its methods now.

Professor Stephen Palmer PhD
Director of the Coaching Psychology Unit, City University,
London, and Director, Centre for Stress Management, UK

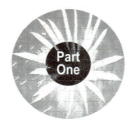

Part
One

Knowledge
is power

Understanding is the first step to control. Accordingly, this part of the book will describe what it means to be out of control, explain the causes, and introduce the solutions available. It will get you started on the road to control by showing you how to identify your needs and decide on strategies.

What does it mean to be out of control?

Control is important to human beings. Since mankind's earliest origins, humans have endeavoured to extend their control over the world around them, and we continue to do so today. Usually, however, we don't consciously think about control until something happens to threaten our sense of being in charge. Ideally, we would react to such a threat with concern and problem-solving behaviour. Unfortunately, it is all too common for people to react with fear: fear of losing their grip over their finances, health, relationships, work and other aspects of their lives.

As well as the practical issues, there is another fear, one that is deeper-seated and often subconscious: that of losing control over oneself. Humans fear their emotions getting out of hand, or they fear losing their mind (or both). This very basic fear is understandable when we consider that if we are not in control of ourselves, then it is unlikely that we will be able to maintain control over our world.

In recent years it has become common, when emotions are intensifying, thoughts are becoming confused and behaviour disorganised, to refer to this state as 'stress'.

Stress has got a bad name. People dislike it. Most view it as something to avoid at any cost. Many people abuse alcohol or drugs to medicate their bad feelings; some use violence to dominate those around them; others act unassertively to avoid the discomfort of disapproval — all of these are attempts to regain control that create new problems of their own.

Stress: a brief introduction

What is this phenomenon that people are so eager to avoid? Until the 20th century, 'stress' was a synonym for 'hardship', 'adversity' and 'affliction'. So, in its older meaning, it referred to *influences on* a person.

About 50 years ago a young doctor named Hans Selye began using the word 'stress' to describe the body's *responses to* various influences on it. Selye saw these responses as the body's way of *adapting* to external influences. His use of the word to include both influences and responses has since entered common usage. Stress is now seen as a process by which the body fights back or attempts to adapt to external influences or challenges. In its modern sense, therefore, the word 'stress' refers to both:

1 the stress *trigger* or 'stressor' — an event or circumstance which you perceive to be a challenge; and

2 the stress *reaction*, consisting of a set of *symptoms* which occur when your entire system gears up to deal with the trigger — physical (for example, your heart speeding up and muscles tightening), emotional (for example, feeling anxiety) and behavioural (for example, getting out of the situation you are in).

Why do human beings feel stress?

You will experience stress when your perception of an event upsets your balance and puts pressure on you to adjust. What goes on in the mind affects the body. The brain sends signals through the nervous system, telling glands to secrete chemicals and muscles to tighten.

Many things can act as stressors, not just negative events but also happy ones — like, for example, getting married. A lack of stimulating events in your life can also be a stressor, by producing the unpleasant need to adjust to boredom. A single event may not be a stressor, but a number of events occurring together can be. Whatever the source, stress occurs when there is a strain on your coping resources.

The origins of the stress response

The stress response is a carry-over from the days when humans were regularly exposed to physical dangers, such as those from wild animals, other hostile humans and food shortages. What we call the 'fight–flight' response — where adrenalin production increases, blood flows to the muscles and breathing speeds up — is designed to prepare the body for physical action. Unfortunately, in modern life this arousal mostly happens in situations that don't call for physical action. Consequently, you are left with your body 'all tensed up and nowhere to go'.

There are three main ways to react to a stressor. You can resist it (the *fight* response), avoid it (the *flight* response) or adapt to it (the *accommodate* response). Each of these reactions can be functional or self-defeating, depending on the situation. Note that 'Nature' does not always know best here. Our bodies, unfortunately, often gear up for physical action when this is not required. To have your muscles tighten and your heart speed up may be useful if a wild animal is after you, but is less helpful when someone makes a critical comment in a committee meeting.

Nature and nurture are both involved. There may be, as we shall see later, some inherited predispositions to certain reactions to stress, but these will be overlaid by learning throughout life.

Why some people have more trouble with control

We all react differently to a perceived challenge. Some people get sick, get depressed, become violent, withdraw, or abuse substances. Others can laugh off problems or take them as they come. Why is this?

How we react to a particular challenge depends on how we *perceive* our ability to cope with it, and how we *evaluate* our ability to manage. For instance, I may perceive that I can cope moderately well, and evaluate this as acceptable, and so feel only moderately stressed. Someone else may likewise perceive that they can cope moderately well, but because they think they should be able to cope 'perfectly', they evaluate this as unacceptable and thus become highly stressed. Yet another person may perceive that they won't be able to cope, but because they accept this reality without any belief that they 'should' be able to cope, they are not unduly distressed. Our beliefs about the events and circumstances occurring in our lives play a crucial role in stress control, and it is in this respect that people differ so much.

Some people are predisposed to have more trouble with control over their reactions to life events. These predispositions, as we shall see later, may be both genetically inherited and learned.

The most significant predisposition is beliefs and attitudes. Stress triggers are not distressing unless we perceive them as such. There are only a limited number of physical sensations we can experience, and our body reacts to all stress triggers in much the same way — increased heart rate, breathing and blood pressure. However, there are a great number of ways in which these sensations can be perceived and evaluated. We learn to put different values on different stress triggers, making some positive and some negative.

A convenient way to illustrate how our reactions to events and circumstances are determined by how we think about them is with the famous 'ABC' model developed about 50 years ago by psychologist Albert Ellis.[1] In this model:

1 **A** represents an *activating event* (a stressor) — for example, you are made redundant;

2 **B** represents your *beliefs* about the 'A' — for example, 'This is the end of the world';

3 **C** is the *consequences* (your reaction) — for example, depression.

Is stress always a bad thing?

Stress itself is not the problem. This may sound strange at first, but *some* stress is essential to your survival and happiness. You need it to motivate you and keep you alert. Even when asleep you are slightly stressed. In fact, without some degree of stress you would be dead. Under-stimulation leads to boredom and sometimes depression. Many people actually seek to increase their stress levels by deliberately jumping out of aeroplanes or engaging in other high-risk activities. The question is not whether stress is good or bad in itself, but rather how much, at which times, and under what conditions it is helpful or unhelpful. Helpful stress we will call 'goodstress', and its dysfunctional opposite 'distress'.

Goodstress

Goodstress involves physical sensations, emotions and behaviours that: (1) are moderate rather than extreme; (2) help you solve your problems and cope with life effectively; and (3) are reduced when they are no longer needed. For example, let's say that you are thinking about an upcoming examination. This is your first exam since you left school many years ago. If you feel mildly anxious, and this is just enough to motivate you to study, and the anxiety goes away when you have finished studying for the evening and prepare for bed, then you are experiencing goodstress.

Goodstress occurs when you either perceive that you have the capabilities required to deal with a situation, or perceive that you lack the capability but *evaluate* this deficiency in a rational way. An example would be that you don't have time to adequately study for the examination, and are therefore likely to fail — but you view failure as sad or disappointing, not as proof you are a total failure as a human being.

The mild anxiety that enhances performance, being in love, and the adrenalin-high of exciting activities are examples of goodstress. Goodstress also includes such negative emotional states as concern, irritation, annoyance or disappointment. While these are unpleasant feelings, they are not disabling and, if handled appropriately, can motivate productive action.

Distress

Distress, in contrast, involves extreme levels of emotional upset, self-defeating behaviour and physical complications — ranging from the high anxiety of panic to the low of depression — that (1) hinder you from coping effectively with your problems and (2) carry on beyond the point where they are useful. Using the example above, if you feel so anxious that you can't concentrate on your study, or the anxiety continues after you have finished studying and stops you from sleeping, then you are experiencing distress.

Distress occurs when you perceive that you lack the capabilities required to meet the demands of a situation *and* evaluate this deficiency in self-defeating ways. For example, you see failing the exam as catastrophic or intolerable, think that it should or must not happen to you, and/or believe that it proves something bad about you as a person.

How much stress is good or bad?

How much stress is 'good' and how much is 'bad' varies from person to person. Some people are happy to live a passive life which others would find boring. Many are only happy when they strive to excel or are stretched in various directions. Most are happier in between these two extremes. Generally, we dislike both a total lack of stress and an excess of it.

The good news

Shortly we will see how to manage external stressors, feel better, and strengthen attitudes that contribute to control over your life. First, though, let us note that human beings seem to have some built-in drives that motivate them to strive at coping with life. As Hans Selye has pointed out, 'the aim of life is to continue its existence'.[2]

We want to do more than just survive, however. Most people want to feel good and avoid discomfort. We want to maximise our pleasure and minimise our pain. When we talk about control, are we not talking about handling life in ways that leave us feeling good — and help us avoid feeling bad?

The big question is: How well do we do this? The chances are your answer will be: 'Not as well as I'd like to!' Although we often go about it in unproductive and inefficient ways, the desire to improve oneself and one's circumstances is part of our basic human nature. Showing how you can make this happen and increase control over your mind, body and life is the purpose of this book.

How to use this book

Let us take an advance look at what lies ahead, and see how you can use this book most efficiently to achieve your goal of effective stress management.

Part One will help you understand what stress is, how to recognise its signs and symptoms, what triggers it, and its underlying causes. You will be introduced to ways in which you can identify your own stress and control problems. You will probably want to read this part only once, to gain a general understanding of stress and its origins.

Part Two shows how you can manage stress by first taking control over yourself. This section of the book is very important. When you have control over yourself, you are in a much better position to take control over your external circumstances. Here you will learn about control over your emotions, and, most importantly, how to control what goes on in your mind.

Part Three continues the theme of control over oneself, in particular: healthy living, control of physical tension and getting a good night's sleep. If you have difficulty with any of these, focus on the relevant chapters.

Part Four will show you how to use a number of practical skills to maximise control over your life, including, as far as it is possible, your external circumstances. Topics will include how to control where your life is going, using support, handling other people, keeping balance in your life, getting more done in the time you have available, letting money reduce your stress rather than increase it, coping with change, solving problems, and managing yourself in the workplace.

Not all of these practical strategies will apply to you; and of those that do, some will be more important than others. Accordingly, you will find it helpful to pick out the chapters that are most relevant and concentrate on those.

If you would like to explore any aspect of stress and its management in more detail, at the end of the book you will find a list of professional books and articles relevant to various aspects of stress management.

To summarise:

- Part One may need reading once only.

- Ensure you study Chapters 5 and 6 in detail.

- Spend time on the remainder of the chapters in Parts Two, Three and Four that are relevant to you.

I wish you all the best as you begin your journey from distress to control!

2

What is out of control for you?

To stay in control it is important to be able to recognise when things are beginning to slip, so that you can take action at an early stage. This chapter will help you identify and prepare a list of your stress symptoms and the typical triggers that activate them. With this step, you will be covering the **C** (consequences) and **A** (activating events) of the ABC stress model.

The general signs of stress

There are many different symptoms of stress. As you read through the following lists, write down or mark the items that you think apply to you.

Specific physical symptoms

Stress generally shows in physical symptoms. Probably the most common is *tension*, where various muscles in the body tighten up. You may also become restless, perhaps even excitable, over-alert, keyed-up, or easily startled. Your heart beats faster and your blood pressure goes up. You become short of breath or breathe faster.

It becomes hard to get a good night's sleep. You feel tired and lack energy. You may lose your appetite, or, conversely, eat more than usual. You become irritable, and experience headaches or other pain. Your mouth and throat goes dry, your face gets hot and flushed, you sweat more.

If your stress gets worse, you may feel weak and possibly dizzy, tremble, develop a nervous tic, grind your teeth, need to pass water more frequently, or experience diarrhoea or constipation, indigestion, queasiness in the stomach, or even vomiting.

General health problems

Stress is often associated with an increased likelihood of physical health problems, such as: digestive problems; high blood pressure, strokes, angina and heart attacks; migraine, chronic pain; irritable bowel syndrome, stomach and duodenal ulcers, and ulcerative colitis. You may become more susceptible to colds and influenza; or experience other health problems, such as diabetes, rheumatoid arthritis, allergies, cancer, asthma, baldness or eczema.

Emotional and cognitive changes

When you are stressed, you will tend to feel and think differently. You will possibly become anxious and worry more than usual. You may find it hard to concentrate, become forgetful, get moody, or feel depressed. You may lose interest or become dissatisfied with your life or your job, feel guilty or down about yourself, feel hostile towards others, or experience other unpleasant emotions.

Behaviours

People usually behave differently when they feel stressed. They may become impatient, short-tempered or aggressive, or in some cases abuse their partner or children.

Stress can lead to impulsive behaviour or hyperactivity, and sometimes even workaholic behaviour where the person would rather keep busy than sleep and feels unhappy when activity stops. Conversely, motivation may be poor; performance goes down, absenteeism increases and there may be procrastination, uncooperativeness, or rebelliousness.

A stressed person might become accident-prone. They may want to cry, run, hide, isolate or withdraw. Stress is often associated with increased smoking, use of prescription drugs (especially tranquillisers), alcohol abuse and illegal drug use.

Concerns expressed by others

Finally, stress may be indicated when other people begin to express concerns. Your partner or children might complain that you are absent, preoccupied or grouchy much of the time; at work, people may comment that you are making more mistakes, or forgetting things; or others remark that your sporting performance has declined.

Special stress conditions

It is wise to be aware of a few conditions that go beyond general stress, so that you can watch for these. Several are, unfortunately, relatively common and require different treatment to general stress.

Burnout

There is a type of stress which, although it can occur in any situation, has been mainly documented in relation to the workplace.[1] Called *burnout,* it is the result of continued and unrelieved stress over a long period.

The typical symptoms are exhaustion, decline in job satisfaction, difficulty coping with role demands, absenteeism, impatience and bad temper, resentment towards colleagues and consumers, and alcohol abuse. It usually progresses in three stages.

In the *early stage*, the person may become over-responsible towards consumers and over-involved with the job (staying late, taking no breaks, avoiding colleagues), and experience minor health problems, such as colds and headaches.

In the *middle stage*, there tends to be a continual negative attitude towards the organisation, with non-constructive complaining to co-workers and blaming of others, occasional inefficiency (for example, slowness, rudeness, forgetfulness), over-compliance, rigid application of rules and instructions, and worsening physical symptoms (such as migraines, influenza, menstrual problems and back-ache).

In the *final stage*, there can be open conflict with the organisation, including tears, rage, hearings, sacking or resignation; an inability to function in the work role, leading to total retreat or paralysis; and worsening physical symptoms, such as nausea, anxiety and stomach problems, which may lead to employment being terminated for medical reasons. Psychiatric referral might occur. The person may renounce their profession or role and retreat to menial tasks or manual work.

Recognising the early signs of burnout will enable you to take corrective action. Prevention, though, is better than cure — if you practise healthy living and good stress management, as described throughout this book, you will stay well away from even the early stages of burnout.

Post-traumatic Stress Disorder (PTSD)

PTSD is a condition that goes beyond generalised stress and is regarded as a diagnosable mental health disorder[2] that may warrant professional intervention.

PTSD may occur following exposure to an unusually traumatic event involving actual or threatened death or serious injury, coupled with intense feelings of fear, horror or helplessness.

The person keeps reliving the event through intrusive and distressing thoughts, images, dreams, flashbacks, hallucinations, illusions or marked distress when reminded of the event. They try to avoid anything that does remind them of the event — feelings, thoughts, conversations, activities, places or people. They may 'forget' aspects of the event or detach themselves from other people. There are symptoms of hyperarousal — such as insomnia, angry outbursts, irritability, poor concentration, excessive vigilance, or increased startle response — that were not present prior to the traumatic event. The symptoms may occur either immediately or at a later stage, and they last longer than one month.

PTSD and its treatment are described in some detail in my book *FearLess*,[3] as are the next two disorders.

Generalised Anxiety Disorder (GAD)

GAD is characterised by excessive worrying about multiple concerns, coupled with a variety of symptoms, such as restlessness, excessive tiredness, poor concentration, irritability, tension and poor sleep. These symptoms will be present most days, for at least six months. Functioning will be affected, although not always severely. See Chapter 7 for detailed information on worrying and how you can get it under control.

Panic disorder

A *panic attack* involves a severe fear or discomfort that peaks within 10 minutes. There are strong symptoms, such as chest pain, chills or hot flashes, a choking feeling, dizziness, heart pounding, nausea, sweating, shortness of breath, trembling, or fears of dying, losing control or going insane.

Panic disorder involves a series of panic attacks coupled with worry about having another attack. They may have a recognisable trigger, although often they do not. Repeated panic attacks usually lead to the person avoiding situations that have come to be associated with the attacks.

Major depression

Depression is one of the most common disorders for which people seek help. It is characterised by (1) lowered mood, or (2) loss of interest or pleasure, or (3) both; coupled with at least three or four of the following:

- appetite or weight changes

- sleep disturbance

- fatigue

- being speeded up or slowed down

- guilt

- poor concentration

- death wishes or suicidal ideas.

These symptoms will be present most of the day, most days, for at least two weeks. Functioning is usually impaired, sometimes quite severely.

Assessing your own stress reactions

If you think that any of the clinical conditions described in the previous section apply to you, consider seeing your doctor or another health professional for a formal assessment.

For most people reading this book, the general stress symptoms listed at the beginning of this chapter will be the focus of their attention. By now you will have made a list of those symptoms you think apply to you. By being aware of these, you can use them as alarm signals that stress is increasing. Then you can take action before things get out of hand. As we shall see later in the book, knowing yourself is a helpful step to effectively managing your stress.

What triggers your stress?

Now it is time to turn to an examination of the events and circumstances that tend to set off your stress response. This represents the **A** (activating events) of the ABC stress model. Knowing what you typically react to will help you identify things you can watch for, and, in some cases, take action to change.

Below is a list of the most common stress triggers. In the next chapter, we will examine what it is within human beings that determines how they react to those triggers. Note down any items in the following list that you think are relevant to you, and also add any unlisted items that come to mind.

Family problems
Marital problems, difficult children, a problem drinker in the family, violence, and the lonely demands of solo parenting can all be triggers for distress in family settings.

Workplace problems
Employees may be distressed when there is a lack of power, too much work or too little, or under- or over-promotion, when authority does not match responsibilities, objectives or requirements are unclear, or there is conflict between multiple job demands, inadequate training, a poor physical working environment, irregular hours of work, sexual harassment, or low job security.

Managers and executives have problems when they find it hard to delegate, their staff are incompetent or poorly trained, they themselves lack control and certainty, or are not used to a participation model and perceive that their power and authority have been stripped.

Being in the wrong job can be distressful — for example, when a high-energy, risk- and stimulation-loving person is in a boring, repetitive job, or a low-energy, safety-conscious person is in a high-flying job.

Lifestyle changes

Any change — even positive change — can be distressful. This may include such events as moving house, starting or finishing your education, marriage, having children, divorce, a new job or different type of work, promotion and retirement. A negative change, such as becoming un-employed, may involve a fear of never again getting meaningful work, financial problems, and loss of status and self-regard.

Developmental changes

Progression through the various phases of the life-cycle brings new stress triggers. Moving from childhood into adolescence means pressures to conform to peers, engage in sexual activity, take drugs, perform educationally, handle conflicts with parents, develop a body image and sex-role identity, and achieve independence from parents.

Middle age involves coping with adolescents, dependent elderly parents, and a growing realisation that some aspirations may never be fulfilled.

Old age may mean enforced retirement, lack of status, failing health, and financial insecurity.

Societal stresses

In the modern world, women are expected to be less emotional and more businesslike; men, more sensitive and in touch with their emotions. Adjusting to these and other changing gender roles can result in conflict and confusion about identity. Throughout the world, there are growing pressures for the recognition of minority groups. The stresses of adaptation to a newly bicultural society in New Zealand, for example, is mirrored in other countries as different cultures strive to take account of each other.

Discrimination may be a stressor: to be picked out on the basis of race, age or sex can mean harassment and difficulty getting work or obtaining finance.

Pressure to achieve status
Stress is often triggered through internal and external demands for high performance, possession of consumer items or a fashionable appearance, or academic, material or sporting success.

Environmental stressors
Increasing migration to city living means adapting to traffic, pollution, noise, crime and isolation. On the other hand, there are stresses for people in rural situations: distance from medical, educational and other services; isolation from other people; a downturn in many rural economies, with post offices and other facilities closing.

Noise can be a stressor: motor vehicles, aircraft, factories, music, the telephone, television sets and stereos are all sources of noise that can create strain.

The mobility that characterises modern society, while advantageous in some respects, can also be a stressor. People increasingly live away from the support of their extended families. The members of some occupational groups, such as police officers and bank officials, have to change their circle of friends regularly.

Technology may be both a blessing and a curse. The increasing pervasiveness of high-tech communications means that bad news spreads rapidly. Television exposes people to constant advertising and violence, and leads to lack of exercise for body and brain, and often boredom. Improvements in transport mean long car journeys, constant danger, fear of flying, and the need to make rapid adjustments to changes in time zone, climate and culture. The availability and convenience of e-mail means that people expect to receive faster responses to their communications.

Then there is commerce. People move between jobs more frequently than in previous eras. Planned obsolescence and high-pressure advertising are increasing factors of modern life.

Positive events

Even supposedly happy events, such as being in love, getting married, having children, being promoted or moving to a better house, can act as triggers for stress.

Internal stress triggers

Internal events are just as likely to act as stress triggers. Physical illness stresses the body — either temporarily, as with a cold or influenza; or longer-term where there is a major illness, disfigurement or disability. People may also react to passing changes in body function, such as the heart missing a beat or a bout of indigestion.

How do external events trigger internal stress?

Stress triggers operate at more than one level. There are *major events* such as natural disasters, accidents, war, imprisonment, divorce and bereavement. More common are the *daily hassles* — an overload of responsibilities, arguments with one's partner, missing the bus, being criticised, and so on.

One or a few challenging events, especially daily hassles, will often not be distressful; but a number that accumulate or coincide may be significant. When a number of stressors have built up, you may react to some supposedly trivial event in a way that surprises you and others — the 'straw that broke the camel's back'. As noted before, even positive events may lead to distress when you get too many of them at once.

Remember, though: *events and circumstances are not distressful unless you perceive and evaluate them as such.* What is distressful to one person may be exciting and stimulating to another. While there are *major events* to which most people react with distress, there are still variations between people in the level and duration of that distress. When it comes to *daily hassles*, there can be an even greater variety of responses from individual to individual.

Identify your top stress triggers

Make a list of your top five stress triggers and place them in order of their significance to you. This personal inventory will serve some useful purposes. You can see if there are any patterns. Do you tend to react to particular people, or in certain situations, or when you are in certain moods? Analyse how you typically feel and behave in response to those triggers. Use your reactions as warning signs that it is time to take action.

To more accurately identify your triggers (activating events) and reactions (consequences), you may find it useful to record, for a few weeks or months, a diary of **A**s and **C**s like the example shown at the top of the next page.

Once you are clear about the **A**s and **C**s in your life, you will be ready to develop and rehearse appropriate coping strategies, such as assertiveness and relaxation. This will prepare you to handle the people or situations to which you typically react, and to control dysfunctional states such as tension or hostility before they get out of hand.

A–C Diary (sample)

A — Activating event	C — Consequence
Manager criticised me in front of team.	Felt hurt all day, concentration down, slow doing my work.
Kids fighting while I was trying to prepare dinner.	Felt angry, yelled at them.

When you are able to effectively manage yourself, you can then set about changing the triggers that are open to change — and accepting the ones that are not.

Why does it happen?

So far you have learned about activating events (**A**s) and their consequences (**C**s). This is not the whole picture, because *external* events and circumstances do not themselves cause *internal* reactions in human beings. We know this because different people experience different reactions to the same trigger. This chapter will explain why, and help you find out why you react as you do to the activating events in your life.

Nature and nurture

A common question people ask is: 'Are we the products of our genetic inheritance, or are we more influenced by environmental factors, including our learning experiences from childhood onwards?' The answer is that both are involved.

Nature: your biochemistry

There is growing evidence that biological make-up plays a part in how people respond to life events.[1] The temperament you are born with will affect, to some degree, how active you are, how you adapt, how intensely you react to things, whether your mood tends to be positive or negative, and how persistent you are.[2]

It appears that some people are more likely to react to things that happen in their environment, and the feelings they experience are more intense. This 'high arousability', as it is called, shows in a variety of ways, such as competitiveness or a tendency to worry, or in clinical conditions, such as generalised anxiety, phobias and obsessive-compulsiveness.

Type A or Type B?

An example of high arousability is the so-called 'Type A' personality. These are people who tend to secrete more adrenalin when under pressure.[3]

People who fit into the Type A category are more likely to possess characteristics regarded as special risk factors for distress, such as the following:

- They feel driven to succeed and fear failure excessively.

- They are highly competitive.

- They tend to overreact to any real or perceived loss of control by becoming highly emotional, and either strive to get control or give up when frustrated.

- They are prone to becoming hostile and aggressive toward others (this may be hidden and be expressed in competitiveness).

- They prefer work to recreation and socialising, and tend to feel guilty when on holiday or when they are not working.

- They tend to feel tense, restless, impatient and irritable, especially when things seem to be happening slowly.

- They often have a sense of being highly pressured by time and what has to be done, are always rushing around, doing everything rapidly; and find it hard to be still.

These tendencies often lead to such problems as sleep disturbance, indigestion, increased risk of heart disease,[4] and difficulties with relationships both in and out of work.

The characteristics described above are in contrast to the 'Type B' personality. These people are more easygoing, less competitive, and not so concerned with failure or loss of control. Type B people can be just as ambitious, work just as hard, and be in equally stressful environments, but they tend to suffer fewer of the harmful effects of stress.

These 'types' are, of course, generalisations. In reality, most people will fit somewhere between the two. Type A traits are more frequently seen in leaders, executives and senior managers. In the past, they were more likely to apply to men, although this is changing as more women enter management positions and ideas about women's roles continue to change. This does not mean that Type A personality characteristics are simply a result of cultural learning — it is more likely that they combine culture *and* biology.

You are not a helpless victim

The fact that there is a biological aspect to our stress problems does not mean that things are hopeless. It simply emphasises the need for hard work to overcome tendencies which may be basic to one's personality. Although it is not possible with our present state of knowledge to permanently change a person's biochemical make-up, what we can do is change faulty learning and develop strategies to compensate for unhelpful aspects of our biological inheritance.

I have seen many people make significant changes in their typical ways of responding to life by learning how to change self-defeating attitudes and develop self-help techniques.

Nurture: the lessons we learn

This brings us to the second aspect of causation. There is more to your personality than biochemistry: environment is also involved.[5] Your biological inheritance is built on by learning from the moment you are born. A biological tendency to high arousability, for example, might be exaggerated by continually trying to avoid uncomfortable feelings ('self-teaching'), or, conversely, it could be minimised by astute parents who teach a child how to manage their arousability.

The most important area of learning concerns the beliefs and attitudes that we take on as children and which, to some extent, we carry with us throughout our lives.

Who do you think controls you?

A key area of your belief system — one that will significantly affect how you react to what life throws at you — is where you think control over yourself is located (your 'locus of control').

If you believe that you have control over your feelings, and at least partial control over the events that shape your life, then you have an *internal* locus of control. You are less likely to experience distress than a person with an *external* locus of control; such individuals see themselves as directed by outside forces — for example, luck, chance, fate , 'the system', or other powers beyond their personal control.[6]

People who have an *external* locus of control typically act and react in a number of ways that increase their risk of distress.[7] They tend, for example, to talk of 'unfairness' or 'unjustness' and view themselves as 'victims'. They are inclined to fear death, both their own and that of people close to them. They become overly distressed when exposed to unwanted events or circumstances. They have a low resistance to infectious diseases, are more susceptible to illness, show the effects of ageing at an early stage, and die younger. After surgery or ill health, they recover slowly, tend to avoid their usual activities for long periods, and trust recovery to luck. They are prone to depression, inclined to choose activities involving luck more than skill, tend to have a low achievement level, and fail to engage in problem-solving behaviour to change circumstances they dislike.

Self-image or discomfort: which bothers you most?

Exactly how do people become emotionally distressed? This can happen in two ways: (1) when they perceive a threat to their self-image, or (2) when they believe that their comfort is at risk; both may also occur together. In either case, the perception of threat is followed by some kind of negative evaluation, either of oneself or of the world.

Self-image disturbance

If you have trouble accepting yourself, you may experience *self-image or 'ego' anxiety*. This is the emotional tension or stress you feel when you believe that your 'self' or personal worth is threatened, or that you must perform well or be approved by others. It is usually accompanied by feelings of inadequacy, guilt, shame or depression.

As well as creating stressful feelings, self-image disturbance leads to self-defeating *behaviours*. If you are overly concerned with status, approval and disapproval, you might act unassertively because you fear what others might think if you ask for what you want or say 'no' to what you don't. Fear of self-downing might cause you to deny — to yourself as well as others — unhelpful characteristics you would be better to change. If you don't trust your own judgement, you will find it hard to make decisions or take risks. And, to complicate things, self-downing may create a block to using many stress-management strategies. If you worry about your appearance, you might, for example, use fad diets rather than eat healthy food, or avoid going to the gym because you think others will laugh at you.

What causes people to overreact when they perceive a threat to their self-image? As we have seen in earlier chapters, the mere perception of a threat will not by itself create distress. Rather, it is the evaluation placed on the perception that determines the reaction. Self-image distur- bance results from two types of evaluative thinking. The first is some kind of belief about the kind of person you *should* be (usually something other than what you are!). Such a 'demand' originates with the normal human tend- ency to want to improve oneself. This preference probably has an evolutionary origin because it increases one's chances of survival. It becomes a problem only when the *preference* for self-improvement is exaggerated into a rigid *demand*.

The second component of self-image disturbance is the tendency to globally evaluate one's whole person. The demands we place on ourselves are often followed by such total self-evaluation. We can illustrate this with the example, introduced in Chapter 1, of preparing for an examination. Let's say you believe that to feel OK about yourself you 'must' always succeed at anything important to you. If you fail the examination, you would then be likely to evaluate or rate yourself as 'useless'. The thinking would be something along these lines: 'I *should* have been able to pass that exam; so because I failed, this shows that *I am a total failure.*' This total, global evaluation of yourself constitutes what is known as 'self-rating'.

Where does this type of thinking come from? Probably, from many years of learning. You may have been told time and time again that you should be better than you are. You may have observed and modelled yourself on a parent who was never satisfied with themself. Perhaps you had experiences while growing up that you interpreted as proof of your badness or uselessness as a person. Consequently, your inherent (and functional) *desire* to continually improve yourself has become a rigid (and dysfunctional) *demand*, which you are never able to satisfy.

Discomfort disturbance

The second type of disturbance occurs when you perceive a threat to your physical or emotional comfort, and then evaluate this threat in some highly negative way. This results in *discomfort anxiety*. It too has demands at its core: the belief that frustration and discomfort 'must' be avoided, coupled with evaluations of these feelings as 'awful' or 'intolerable'.

Whereas in self-image disturbance the demands and evaluations are directed inwards at oneself, in discomfort disturbance they are directed outwards. In effect, we tell ourselves that the world around us 'must' be a certain way, otherwise it will be 'awful' or 'unbearable'. If you *perceive* that your comfort (or life) is threatened, then *evaluate* this as 'unbearable' (rather than disadvantageous), and tell yourself that it 'must' not happen (instead of preferring that it not occur), then you will become distressed.

Discomfort disturbance expresses itself in two main ways. *Low frustration tolerance* occurs when a person views frustration as 'catastrophic' and believes that it 'should' not happen to them. *Low discomfort tolerance* results from exaggerating the badness of such things as physical pain, negative emotions and loss of lifestyle, coupled with the demand that these things 'must' be avoided. Like self-image disturbance, discomfort disturbance leads to both distressful emotions and self-defeating behaviours:

- *Worrying* is the result of evaluating certain events or circumstances as 'awful' or 'unbearable', which leads to the idea that we 'must' worry about them in case they happen.

- *Avoidance* of discomfort also results from evaluating events and circumstances catastrophically.

- *Short-range enjoyment* leads people to seek immediate pleasure or avoidance of pain, at the cost of long-term stress. It shows in such behaviours as abuse of alcohol, drugs and food; watching television at the expense of exercising; practising unsafe sex; or overspending to feel better.

- *Procrastination.* Short-range enjoyment and the avoidance of discomfort may lead to putting off difficult tasks or unpleasant situations — which leads to more stress in the long run.

- *Addictive tendencies.* Low discomfort tolerance is a key factor in the development of addictions.[8] To resist the impulse of the moment, and go without, will be uncomfortable or frustrating; if the discomfort is rated as 'awful' or 'unbearable', then it will seem easier to give in to the urge to misuse alcohol, take drugs, gamble or exercise obsessively. Much addictive behaviour serves to help people avoid pain: substance abusers are, in effect, medicating themselves to get rid of bad feelings. Unfortunately, once this tendency is established, it is hard to give up. Quite apart from damage to the body and strained relationships, addictive behaviour can mean a significant loss of control.

- *Victimhood.* Low discomfort tolerance may lead a person to become distressed over small hindrances and setbacks, overly concerned with unfairness, and prone to make comparisons between their own and others' circumstances. Seeing oneself as a victim of injustice is almost like handing over control of one's emotions, sometimes to the very people seen as the perpetrators.

Four ways to upset yourself: evaluative thinking

The preceding discussion of self-image and discomfort disturbance reiterates an important idea introduced in Chapter 1; namely, that distress results not just from *perceiving* that you lack the ability to cope with something, but more particularly from *evaluating* that lack in certain negative ways. There are four types of evaluative thinking that typically contribute to distress: 'demandingness' (applicable to both types of disturbance), 'awfulising' and 'can't-stand-it-itis' (relevant to discomfort disturbance), and 'self-rating' (associated with self-image disturbance).

1 *Demandingness*. When you think in terms of rigid 'shoulds' and 'musts', you place demands on yourself, other people and the world. There are two main types: *moralising* — using words like 'should' or 'ought' (for example, 'I should be able to pass this examination'); and *musturbation* — thinking that things 'must', 'need' or 'have to' be certain ways (for example, 'I *must* (or *need to* or *have to*) pass this examination'). Demands create an internal feeling of pressure and escalate stress reactions. They often, also, have a paradoxical effect. For example, if you believe that you absolutely 'must' have control over your feelings and actions, you will make yourself so anxious that you increase the chance of losing control! Demandingness contributes to both self-image and

discomfort disturbance. To rate your total self indicates that you are (probably at a subconscious level) comparing yourself with some kind of standard that is held as a rigid, absolute demand, like: 'To be a worthwhile human being, I *should* be able to succeed at anything important I try — so, because I failed the exam, *I* must be useless.' The subconscious demand to succeed comes first; the self-rating of 'useless' derives from it and leads to self-image disturbance.

The same process operates with discomfort disturbance. If you hold a demand about security, safety, avoidance of pain or experiencing negative feelings, then when you are faced with the situation you believe 'must' not happen, you will evaluate it catastrophically. For example, 'Because I *must* not experience pain, etc, it would be *awful* or *unbearable* if it happened.' Note, too, that the process can operate in reverse: if you catastrophise about something, then you are more likely to demand that it must not happen. The potential for a vicious circle of thinking will no doubt be obvious.

2 *Awfulising.* If you exaggerate the badness of future events and circumstances (for example, 'It would be *dreadful* to fail this examination') then you are 'awfulising'. Typical awfulising words are 'terrible', 'horrible' and the like. Seeing things as worse than they really are escalates stressful feelings and leads to self-defeating avoidance behaviour. Awfulising is a key factor in discomfort disturbance.

3 *Can't-stand-it-itis.* Evaluating events and experiences as 'unbearable' has a similar effect to awfulising. The two often mix with each other and with demandingness — for example, 'It would be *dreadful* and *unbearable*

to fail this examination, so I *must* not fail.' Can't-stand-it-itis contributes to discomfort disturbance.

4 *Self-rating*. Evaluating or 'rating' your actions — for example, 'I failed this exam' — is useful because it enables you to learn from experience and improve your functioning. Unfortunately, however, it is all too common to jump from rating the action to rating the *entire self:* for example, 'I failed this exam — therefore *I* am a failure'; thus creating self-image disturbance.

Perceptions: they are not always accurate

As well as evaluating events and circumstances in self-defeating ways, it is also possible to misperceive them in the first place. For instance, you may think that you lack the ability to pass the examination, but this perception may be incorrect. You could be basing it on the fact that when you were at school you failed some important examinations, and recalling this leads you to think that you are 'always' failing and always will. This is a type of misperception known as 'over-generalising'.

Perceptions are sometimes also referred to as 'interpretations' or 'inferences'. They represent *supposedly* 'factual' statements about what has happened, is happening, or might happen. Faulty perceptions represent conclusions about a situation that are drawn prematurely, without a full understanding of the situation. There are seven ways in which we might misinterpret events and circumstances, shown in the table on the next page.

Core beliefs

Sitting underneath perceptions and evaluations of *specific* events and circumstances are our *general* 'core beliefs'.

Seven ways to misperceive events and circumstances

Type of perception	Example
Black-and-white thinking Viewing things in extremes, with no middle ground.	'Because I didn't get through all the material, my presentation was a total waste of time for the staff.'
Filtering Seeing all that is wrong, while ignoring (filtering out) the positives.	'There's nothing good about this restructuring.'
Over-generalising Assuming one event or circumstance represents the total situation.	'Everything's going wrong in my life.'
Mind-reading Jumping to a conclusion, without evidence, about what other people are thinking.	'She did it because she hates me.'
Fortune-telling Treating beliefs about the future as realities rather than just predictions.	'We'll end up in debt now that overtime has been cut.'
Emotional reasoning Believing that because you *feel* a certain way, this is how it really is.	'I just know things are going to go badly, because I feel so anxious.'
Personalising Jumping to the conclusion, without evidence, that you are responsible for something.	'It's because I am so slow that the whole team won't be getting a pay rise this year.'

Everyone has a set of beliefs and attitudes, mostly in the form of 'rules for living'. They are general in the sense that they may apply to a range of situations. They are reasonably enduring — we learn most of them in childhood, and in some form or other they may persist throughout our lives. Our core beliefs are with us all the time, although because they are held subconsciously we are not usually aware of them. Most of them are quite rational and aid our day-to-day functioning; it is only a few that are disadvantageous to us.

The 12 self-defeating core beliefs

Psychologist Albert Ellis, one of the early originators of the method of psychotherapy now known as 'Cognitive Behaviour Therapy', has suggested that most self-defeating core beliefs are variations of one or other of a small list of key ideas. Here is a slightly expanded and modified version of his list:

1 I need to get love and approval from the people who are significant to me, and I must avoid disapproval from any source.

2 To be worthwhile as a person I must achieve, succeed at whatever I do, and make no significant mistakes.

3 People should always do the right thing. When they behave obnoxiously, unfairly or selfishly, they must be blamed and punished.

4 Things must be the way I want them to be, otherwise life will be intolerable.

5 My unhappiness is caused by things outside my control, so there's little I can do to feel any better.

6 I must worry about things that could be dangerous, unpleasant or frightening, otherwise they might happen.

7 I can be happier by avoiding things that are difficult or unpleasant.

8 Everyone needs to depend on someone stronger than themselves.

9 Events in my past are the cause of my problems, and they continue to influence my feelings and behaviours now.

10 I should become upset when other people have problems, and feel unhappy when they're sad.

11 I shouldn't have to feel discomfort and pain. I can't stand them and must avoid them at all costs.

12 Every problem should have an ideal solution, and it's intolerable when one can't be found.

Everyone has their own set of beliefs. Consider the list above: which of these beliefs do you sense might be operating for you? It is your own system of core beliefs that determines how you perceive and evaluate what happens to you. To take greater control over yourself and your life, you need to learn how to identify and change those core beliefs that are dysfunctional. How to do that is a topic we will come to shortly.

Putting it all together

As we have seen, your biological inheritance and past learning sets the scene, but what determines how you react to stress triggers in the present are the beliefs you carry with you now. Once you know how to identify and change self-defeating beliefs, you will know how to regain and retain control. The first step is knowing what to look for, and you have taken that step by studying this chapter. Here's a summary of the material we have covered.

In Chapter 2 you examined your activating events and consequences (the **A** and **C** of the ABC stress model). In the present chapter you filled in the gap and studied the **B** (beliefs) part.

How you react (**C**) to a stress trigger (**A**) will depend, largely, on how you view it (**B**). To experience stress, you would need to perceive an event or circumstance as a threat to your physical or emotional comfort, self-image, or lifestyle; and as a challenge to your ability to cope. If you *perceive* that you can cope, you will most likely experience *good*stress. If you perceive that you can't cope but *evaluate* this in a functional way (for example, as unfortunate but bearable), you will also experience goodstress.

If, however, you perceive that you can't cope and evaluate this *irrationally* (for example, you tell yourself that you 'have to' cope and that it is 'awful' and 'unbearable' that you cannot), then you will experience *dis*tress.

Your assessment may be accurate or it may be distorted. Your coping system might be activated when it does not need to be, because you perceive danger when it does not exist or you overestimate it. (It is also possible to be under-aroused and fail to recognise a real danger — for example, when a person drives after drinking alcohol.)

How you perceive and evaluate life events ultimately depends on the set of core beliefs that you hold. For example, if you hold a core belief like: 'Everything I do must be perfect', then you may be predisposed to worry about and thus exaggerate the likelihood of failure, and evaluate that possibility in a catastrophic fashion.

The ABC model

A convenient way to illustrate the whole process is with the ABC model introduced in Chapter 1. To recap: **A** is the 'activating event' or stress trigger; **B** represents your thoughts and beliefs about the **A**; and **C** is the 'consequence', your reaction. Here's how it works: an event or experience 'activates' one or other of your core beliefs; this shapes your perception of the event and your subsequent evaluation; this then creates your emotional and behavioural consequence.

Here's an example, using the same stressor, with two different ways of thinking about it leading to two very different consequences:

A	Event:	Received a large car repair bill in the mail	
B	Core belief activated:	I can't stand discomfort and must avoid it at all costs.	It is better to face discomfort now than avoid it and suffer more later.
	Perceptions: pay for it.	We don't have the money to pay for it.	We don't have the money to pay
	Evaluations:	This is terrible. I can't bear to think about it.	This is unfortunate. I'd better do something about it.
C	Emotions:	Felt tense and anxious.	Felt concerned.
	Behaviours:	Put the bill away and tried not to think about it.	Telephoned garage and arranged to pay by instalments.

This example illustrates what happens when we react to life events. Fortunately, a negative reaction is not the end of the story. Because thinking is the main cause of how we react, we can reduce our stress by changing what we think. Learning how to do this will be a key focus of the next few chapters.

Three targets for change

By incorporating the three components involved with experiences — triggering event, thoughts and reaction — the ABC model also points to the fact that we have not just one, but three ways in which we can take control:

1 by changing the activating event, when this is possible (for example, by managing finances so the money for car repairs is set aside in advance);

2 by directly changing the consequence — how we feel (for example, by using a tension-relaxation technique); or

3 by changing the **B** — what we tell ourselves in specific stressful situations, and the underlying core beliefs that

repetitively cause us to misperceive those situations and evaluate them in self-defeating ways.

Can we overcome our predispositions?

There are certain things that, with our present state of knowledge, we cannot change. But even when they are part of our genetic inheritance or personality, we can learn how to 'mediate' unhelpful tendencies and thus manage our lives effectively in spite of them. Remember that the main determinant of how you feel and behave is your belief system and what you think about yourself, others, and the world. You can choose to change those beliefs. Neither your inherited nor your learned characteristics have to totally control your life.

Taking control:
first steps

The chapters that follow consist of information that will help you take control over yourself and your life. The strategies presented have been developed from many years of experience helping people with their control issues, and from studying research on stress management from around the world.

At the top of the list of strategies is rational thinking. How you feel and behave is largely determined by how you think, so to take control over *yourself* you need to know how to identify and replace self-defeating thinking. To take control over your *life* you need a range of strategies to manage your health, time, money, other people, work and change — strategies that can be enhanced by rational thinking, or undercut by self-defeating thinking. Accordingly, showing how to develop rational thinking skills will be the overriding focus of this book.

Experience and research indicate there are 12 key strategies that contribute to control over an individual's life. You will already be using some of these strategies; others you may be struggling with. Soon you will have the opportunity to determine which of the strategies is best to spend your time on.

Here is the list:

1 Know where your life is going: have clear and realistic goals.

2 Manage time to achieve your goals.

3 Know how to solve the problems that occur in your life.

4 Be able to sleep well.

5 Take care of your body, what you put into it and how you use it.

6 Be able to relax your body and mind to control tension.

7 Keep balance in your life.

8 Maintain a support system.

9 Be able to handle other people.

10 Manage your financial and material resources.

11 Manage the inevitable changes in your life.

12 Be able to ask for help when you need it.

Find out what you most need to work on

If you have carried out the suggestions for action in preceding chapters, then you will have already assessed your typical stress reactions and listed the most common triggers for these. Next, I recommend that you complete the *Life Control Options Questionnaire* given in the Extras at the back of the book. This will help you identify those areas you will probably benefit most from working on.

A key point: management, not cure

It is understandable to hope that once you have achieved control you will be cured for life and will never have to combat stress again. Unfortunately, such an idea will only lead to disillusionment, because problems and stress are part of the human condition. What you are going to do is learn some skills which, for the rest of your life, you can use as required.

Personal control involves using strategies to help you function better in everyday life and influence what happens to you. Although these strategies will become more habitual as time goes by, you will still need to use them, often consciously and deliberately, throughout your life. If you adopt the approach of management rather than cure, you will almost certainly be able to maintain control in the long term.

Attend to the triggers, the consequences and the attitudes

Good management involves taking action on both your internal reactions and the external triggers. But most importantly, it involves dealing with the beliefs that come between the two and ultimately determine how you feel and behave. This book will show you how to deal with all three.

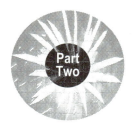

Part
Two

Control
over your mind
and emotions

In Part One the focus was on understanding the causes of distress and identifying your own stress reactions and their triggers. Now it is time to move from the problem to the solution; in other words, from understanding to action. The rest of this book is committed to helping you gain the skills that will enable you to manage yourself and your world. We will begin with the most important area of all, the essential prerequisite to control over your life: managing what goes on in your mind when you face life and what it throws at you.

What is rational thinking?

To manage our lives, we first need to manage ourselves. This involves knowing how to identify the self-defeating beliefs that create unnecessary distress and change them to more helpful ways of thinking. That raises the question: when you get rid of an old, dysfunctional way of thinking, what do you replace it with? This chapter will define rational thinking, outline rational alternative modes or types of thinking, then finish with an extended listing of rational principles from which you can draw as you seek to change the content of those beliefs you identify as causing you unnecessary strife.

Self-defeating versus rational thinking

We'll begin with two definitions — one of self-defeating thinking, the other of rational thinking — looking at them side-by-side for comparison.

A self-defeating belief:	A rational belief:
is harmful: it creates extreme negative emotions and blocks you from achieving your goals.	*is helpful:* it results in moderate emotions appropriate to a situation and helps you achieve your goals.
is not supported by the evidence.	*is in line with the evidence.*

(Continued)

A self-defeating belief:	A rational belief:
is illogical: – involves rigid demands ('shoulds' and 'musts') – exaggerates the badness of events and circumstances – rates the whole person instead of just their actions.	*is logical:* – stresses preferential thinking – keeps the badness of things in perspective – judges behaviour, not the person.

Alternative modes of thinking

Now let's see how the definition of rational thinking works out in practice.

Below is an outline of the 'modes' or types of self-defeating thinking described in Chapter 3, with the rational alternative to each.

New perceptions

Here are alternatives to the seven ways in which we mis-perceive events and circumstances:

Black-and-white thinking	Replace with 'continuum' thinking that reflects the reality that things are rarely completely one way or another.
Filtering	Replace with thinking that takes into account both negatives and positives.
Over-generalising	To get things into perspective, identify just how often a negative experience really is occurring.
Mind-reading	Accept that you may not know what is in someone else's mind, and look for alternative explanations for their behaviour, other than the first conclusion that sprang into your mind.
Fortune-telling	Treat a belief about the future as simply a prediction and nothing more. Examine the evidence and establish the real likelihood of your prediction coming true.

(Continued)

Emotional reasoning	Remind yourself that your emotions are caused by your own thinking — not the situation — and that sometimes your thinking may not be accurate.
Personalising	Look for alternative possible explanations for something that has happened, other than the conclusion that you are to blame, then examine the evidence for each one.

New evaluations

Each of the four types of evaluative thinking has a rational substitute:

Demandingness ('should', 'must', 'need', etc)	Replace with a preference ('prefer', 'would be better', 'desirable', etc).
Awfulising ('awful', 'terrible', etc)	Replace with 'bad', 'unpleasant', 'uncomfortable'.
Can't-stand-it-itis ('unbearable', 'can't stand', etc)	Replace with 'endurable', 'I don't like', etc.
Self-rating ('I am ...')	Replace with 'I do ...' (rate your behaviour, not yourself).

The 12 rational principles

The thinking patterns described above concern 'types' or 'modes' of thinking — for example, demanding versus preferring, self-rating versus behaviour-rating, and so on. But what does the *content* of rational thinking look like?

The 12 principles outlined in the following section provide some key examples of content. They represent a summary of my research over many years into what constitutes rational thinking, in terms of the definition at the start of this chapter. This material has been culled both from the literature on cognitive behaviour therapy and from my own years of experience of working on my own disturbances and helping my clients overcome theirs.

1 Know yourself

Self-knowledge is not, strictly speaking, an example of rational thinking so much as something you actually *do*. However, the other principles build on it, as do many of the self-help strategies you will meet in other chapters, so we begin with it.

Self-knowledge involves knowing your capabilities and your limits, your personal temperament and typical coping style, and your values and goals:

- What are your values? What matters to you? While you may share many ideals with others in your social group, every person has a unique system of values and goals.

- Everyone has certain abilities — and limits. Do you recognise your abilities and make the most of them? Do you also acknowledge your limits and know when to stop?

Everyone has their own temperament, style of managing stress, and value system. For coping strategies to be effective, you need to develop those that are relevant to your personal style and compatible with your personal values; otherwise, you are not likely to use them.

Completing the *Life Control Options Questionnaire* (in the Extras section at the back of the book) is one way to increase your knowledge of yourself.

2 Accept yourself and have confidence in your abilities

To *accept yourself* is to acknowledge three things: (1) you exist; (2) there is no reason why you *should* be any different from how you are; and (3) you are neither worthy nor unworthy.

Self-acceptance involves rejection of any *demand* that you be different. You may sensibly *prefer* to be different and decide to change some things. But you are best to keep the desire to change as a preference — you don't *have* to change, it is a *choice*.

Further, instead of evaluating your *'self'*, use your energy and time to evaluate (1) your *behaviour,* and (2) the quality of your *existence*. Evaluating your behaviour is a good idea: you can monitor how effective it is in helping you enjoy your life and achieve your goals. It is also a good idea to evaluate the quality of your existence: your enjoyment of life is surely important — more important than worrying about whether you are a 'worthwhile' person.

Self-acceptance is not the same thing as the commonly held (but misguided) notion of 'self-esteem' — which represents self-rating, albeit in a positive direction. *Self-esteem* is based on the idea that you are a 'good' or 'worthwhile' person. Unfortunately, worthwhileness requires criteria, like how well you perform (which means you become 'not worthwhile' when your performance is not up to scratch!), or some underpinning philosophical concept like the vague and unprovable idea that you are, somehow, worthwhile simply because you exist (a tricky concept: the smart person will realise that if we can be worthwhile just because we exist, then, equally, we can be worthless because we exist!).

Self-acceptance, on the other hand, is based on the idea that you don't *have* to be 'good' or 'worthwhile'. In fact, there is no need to evaluate your*self* at all! Instead of evaluating your 'self' (whatever that means), you use your energy and time to evaluate your *behaviour* and the quality of your *existence*.

Similarly, rather than striving for 'self-confidence', aim instead to have *confidence in your abilities*. This involves three things. First, you acknowledge what you can and can't do. Secondly, you are prepared to try things to the limit of your ability. And thirdly, you regularly work at extending your capabilities.

Having confidence in your *abilities* is different to having confidence in your *self*. 'Self'-confidence implies perfection — that you, as a *total* person, are able to do everything well. Confidence in your *abilities* is more realistic. Instead of talking about *self*-confidence, aim for *ability*-confidence[1] and talk about social confidence, work confidence, driving confidence, house-care confidence, examination confidence, relationship confidence, and so on.

For more information on self-acceptance and specific strategies that can help you achieve it, see page 80.

3 Practise enlightened self-interest

It is important to your survival and happiness that you are able to act in your own interests. It is also important to take into account the interests of others. The principle of enlightened self-interest takes both of these views into account: (1) your own interests are placed first; while (2) you keep in mind that your own interests will be best served if you also consider the interests of others.

In other words, ensure your self-interest is *enlightened*. *Individual* interests are best served by *mutual* cooperation. Self-interest without social interest is misguided; so is social interest without self-interest. Knowing what is in your interests will help you get what is best for you and avoid what is harmful, and keep you moving towards your goals.

You had better also take into account the interests of others: treat other people well and they are more likely to reciprocate. Contribute to their welfare and they will be encouraged to contribute to yours. And contributing to the society in which you live will mean a better environment in which to pursue your interests.

4 Tolerate frustration and discomfort

High tolerance will keep you from overreacting to things you dislike. It will help you tackle problems and issues rather than avoid them. It will enable you to take risks and try new experiences. 'High tolerance' means accepting the reality of frustration and discomfort, and keeping the badness of events and circumstances in perspective.

To accept frustration and discomfort is to acknowledge that, while you may dislike them, they are realities. They exist, and there is no law of the universe to say they 'should' not exist (although you might *prefer* they did not). You expect to experience *appropriate* negative emotions, such as concern, remorse, regret, sadness, annoyance and disappointment. But you avoid exaggerating these emotions (by telling yourself you can't stand them) into anxiety, guilt, shame, depression, hostile anger, hurt or self-pity. There are suggestions for raising discomfort tolerance in the next chapter.

5 Enjoy the present and the future

Like most people, you probably want to enjoy life. As well as avoiding distress, you want to experience pleasure. And you probably want to get your pleasure now, not tomorrow. But there are times when it is in our interests to forgo immediate pleasure in order to have greater enjoyment in the longer term. Accordingly, operate on the principle of *long-range enjoyment.*

Seek to get satisfaction from each of your present moments, rather than always putting off pleasure until 'tomorrow' (or dwelling on things that have happened in the past). However, to keep on enjoying your present moments, choose to postpone pleasure at times. You may wish to drink more alcohol — but if you restrict your intake now your body will still let you drink in 10 years' time. Or you may wish to buy a new stereo, but instead choose to save the money for an overseas trip.

To sum up: *live for the present with an eye to the future.* Seek to get maximum pleasure and enjoyment in the present, while ensuring you will be able to enjoy life in the long term.

6 *Take (sensible) risks*

Human beings, by nature, seek safety, predictability, and freedom from fear. But humans also pursue risk. A totally secure life would be a boring one. To grow as a person and improve your quality of life means being prepared to take some chances.

Be willing to take sensible risks in order to get more out of life and avoid the distress of boredom, listlessness and dissatisfaction. Learn new things that may challenge existing beliefs; tackle tasks that have no guarantee of success; try new relationships; do things even though there is a risk that others may disapprove.

7 *Be moderate in all things*

Sensible risk-taking recognises that human beings also desire safety and security. The principle of moderation will help you avoid extremes in thinking, feeling and behaving.

Extreme expectations that are too high or too low will set you up for either constant failure or a life of boredom. Addictive or obsessional behaviour can take control of you. Unrestrained eating, drinking or exercising will stress your body and lead to long-term health complications. Obsessive habits can damage relationships as well as your body.

Take a moderate approach to your whole life — from your ultimate goals through to your daily activities. Develop long-term goals, short-term objectives, and tasks that will challenge and move you on — while ensuring that they are achievable and do not set you up to become disillusioned. Moderation does not exclude risk-taking — in fact, it will help you avoid taking security too far. You don't have to be foolhardy to take risks.

8 Take responsibility for your emotions and behaviours

People who see their emotions and behaviours as under their control are less prone to distress than people who see themselves as controlled by external forces.[2] To be *emotionally responsible* is to believe that you create your own feelings, and you avoid blaming other people or your circumstances for how you feel. *Behavioural responsibility* involves accepting that you cause your own actions and behaviours, and are not compelled to behave in any particular way.

Note that responsibility is not the same thing as blame. 'Blame' is *moralistic* — it seeks to damn and condemn. Responsibility, on the other hand, is *practical*. It seeks either to identify a cause so that this can be dealt with, or to identify who needs to take action for the problem to get solved. It is concerned not with moralising but with finding solutions.

9 Direct your own life and commit to action

Self-direction involves: (1) choosing your goals, making sure they are your own; and (2) making your own decisions, even though you may seek opinions from others. Self-direction does not mean refusing to cooperate with others — you keep it on the right track by balancing it with enlightened self-interest, moderation and flexibility.

Commitment follows from self-direction. It has two elements: perseverance and deep involvement.

- *Perseverance* is the ability to bind yourself emotionally and intellectually to a course of action, and involves a willingness to do the necessary work — and tolerate the discomfort involved — in personal change and goal achievement.

- *Deep involvement* is the ability to enjoy and become absorbed in (but not addicted to) other people, activities and interests — work, sports, hobbies, creative activities and the world of ideas — as ends in themselves, where you get pleasure from the doing, irrespective of the final result.

10 Take a flexible approach to life

Flexible people can bend with the storm rather than be broken by it.

They know how to *adapt* and adjust to new circumstances that call for new ways of thinking and behaving. They have *resilience* — the ability to bounce back from adversity.

Be open to change in yourself and in the world. As circumstances alter, modify your plans and behaviours. Adopt new ways of thinking that help you cope with a changing world. Let others hold their own beliefs and do things in ways appropriate to them, while you do what is right for you.

Be flexible in your *thinking*. Ensure your values are preferences rather than demands. Be open to changing ways of thinking in the light of new information and evidence. View change as a challenge rather than a threat.

Be flexible in your *behaviour*. Change direction when it is in your interests. Try new ways of dealing with problems and frustrations. Let others do things their way, and avoid distressing yourself when they think or act in ways you dislike.

11 Keep your thinking objective

All of the other principles require freedom from ways of thinking that are narrow-minded, sectarian, bigoted and fanatical; or that rely on uncritical acceptance of dogmatic beliefs or 'magical' explanations for the world and what happens in it.

Objective thinking is scientific in nature. It is *empirical*: based on evidence gained from observation and experience rather than on subjective feelings or uncritical beliefs. It is *logical*: conclusions validly follow from the evidence. Most important, it is *pragmatic*: it results in appropriate emotions (*good*stress) and behaviours that help us achieve our goals.

Nothing is seen as absolute or the last word. Beliefs are seen as theories that are subject to change as new evidence comes to hand. Objectivity encourages us to continually search for explanations that are more accurate and useful than the ones we have now.

12 Accept reality

It makes sense, wherever possible, to change things you dislike. But there will be some things you will not be able to change. You then have two choices: you can rail against fate and stay distressed; or you can accept reality and move on. To accept something is to do three things:

1 *Admit that reality — including unpleasant reality — exists*. See it as inevitable that many things will not be to your liking. View uncertainty, frustration and disappointment as aspects of normal life.

2 *Avoid any demand that reality not exist*. This means that although you may *prefer* that yourself, other people, things or circumstances be different from how they are (and you may even work at changing them),

you know there is no law of the universe that says they *should* or *must* be different.

3 *Keep unwanted realities in perspective.* When you dislike something, define it as undesirable and unpleasant — but avoid catastrophising it into 'horrible' or 'unbearable'.

Many people have trouble with the idea of acceptance. They think that to accept something means they have to like it, agree with it, justify it, be indifferent to it, or resign themselves to it. Acceptance is none of these things. You can dislike something, see it as unjustified and continue to prefer that it not exist. You can be concerned about it. You can take action to change it, if change is possible. But you can still accept it by rejecting the idea that it *should* not exist and that it absolutely *must* be changed. To paraphrase a well-known saying: to achieve happiness, you should strive for (1) the courage to change the things you can, (2) the serenity to accept the things you can't, and (3) the wisdom to know the difference.[3]

To see how these principles may be applied to one particular area of life — work and the workplace — read Chapter 20.

One last thing. Don't make these principles into demands: they are ideals. Probably no one could practise them all consistently. Rather than seeing them as absolute 'musts' for managing your life, use them as *guidelines* to a better existence.

The 12 core beliefs: from self-defeat to personal control

To finish our examination of rational thinking, in the left-hand column of the table opposite are the 12 self-defeating core beliefs presented in Chapter 3. Beside each is a rational alternative more likely to facilitate personal control. You may find this a useful checklist to have on hand as you develop the art of formulating new beliefs.

Self-defeating beliefs	Personal control beliefs
I need to get love and approval from the people who are significant to me, and I must avoid disapproval from any source.	Love and approval are good things to have and I'll seek them when I can, but they're not necessities. I can survive (albeit uncomfortably) without them.
To be worthwhile as a person I must achieve, succeed at whatever I do, and make no significant mistakes.	I'll always seek to achieve as much as I can, but unfailing success and competence is unrealistic. Better that I just accept myself as a person, separate from my performance.
People should always do the right thing. When they behave obnoxiously, unfairly or selfishly, they must be blamed and punished.	It's unfortunate that people sometimes do bad things. But humans aren't yet perfect, and upsetting myself won't change that reality.
Things must be the way I want them to be, otherwise life will be intolerable.	There is no law that says things have to be the way I want. It's disappointing, but I can stand it — especially if I avoid catastrophising.
My unhappiness is caused by things outside my control, so there's little I can do to feel any better.	Many external factors are outside my control. But it's my thoughts (not the externals) which cause my feelings, and I can learn to control my thoughts.
I must worry about things that could be dangerous, unpleasant or frightening, otherwise they might happen.	Worrying about things that might go wrong won't stop them happening. It will, however, ensure that I get upset and disturbed right now!
I can be happier by avoiding things that are difficult or unpleasant.	Avoiding problems is only easier in the short term — putting things off can make them worse later on. It also gives me more time to worry about them!

(Continued)

Self-defeating beliefs	Personal control beliefs
Everyone needs to depend on someone stronger than themselves.	Relying on someone else can lead to dependent behaviour. It's OK to seek help, so long as I learn to trust myself and my own judgement.
Events in my past are the cause of my problems, and they continue to influence my feelings and behaviours now.	The past can't influence me now. My current beliefs cause my reactions. I may have learned these beliefs in the past, but I can choose to analyse and change them in the present.
I should become upset when other people have problems, and feel unhappy when they're sad.	It's good to care and help when I can, but I can't change other people's problems and bad feelings by getting myself upset.
I shouldn't have to feel discomfort and pain. I can't stand them and must avoid them at all costs.	Why should I in particular not feel discomfort and pain? I don't like them, but I can stand them. Also, my life would be very restricted if I always avoided discomfort.
Every problem should have an ideal solution, and it's intolerable when one can't be found.	Problems usually have many possible solutions. It's better to stop waiting for the perfect one and get on with the best available. I can live with less than the ideal.

6

How to apply
rational thinking

Now that you know what constitutes rational thinking, the next step is to move from understanding to application. You may, however, be wondering if this is easier said than done. How do you change ways of thinking that you may have held all your life? Fortunately, there are numerous strategies that have been developed to help people do just that.

One such set of procedures is known as *Rational Effectiveness Training* (RET for short), developed by Dr Dominic DiMattia of the Albert Ellis Institute in New York. It is based on rational-emotive behaviour therapy, devised by Albert Ellis in the 1950s, and applies Dr Ellis's methods to stress management and coping effectiveness in a range of areas, including the workplace.[1]

As the previous chapter showed, to cope effectively with modern life you need a rational philosophy for living. You also need to *live according to that philosophy*. New ways of feeling and behaving will not come automatically — but they will come with work and practice.

Rational effectiveness training provides the tools to help you handle distressful emotional states, change self-defeating behaviours, eliminate blocks to applying stress-management strategies, and increase your productivity. The version of RET presented in this book reflects the work of Drs Ellis and DiMattia, along with developments by myself and other practitioners.

A key RET technique: Rational self-analysis

Rational self-analysis is a technique you can use to identify and change the thoughts involved when you experience distress or behave in self-defeating ways. Analysing your thinking can not only help you reduce current distress, but will also decrease the likelihood of repeating the same self-defeating reactions in the future.

Rational self-analysis builds on the 'ABC' model described in earlier chapters. Here is a summary of the procedure:

Identify the *Activating event* — the stress trigger to which you are reacting.

Describe the *Consequence* — the distressful feelings and unhelpful behaviours that comprise your reaction.

Identify the *Beliefs* — what are you thinking about the **A** that is causing your reaction at **C**?

Identify the new *Effect* you want to achieve — how would you prefer to feel and behave differently to the current **C**?

Dispute — question the old beliefs, decide which are self-defeating, and replace those with new beliefs.

Develop *Further action* — what you will do to consolidate the new thinking and reduce the chance of continuing to react in the old way.

An example

Here is an example of a rational self-analysis to show how it works in practice. Carol, a team leader in the local office of a large government department, was criticised by her boss within the hearing of other staff. For the rest of the day Carol was very emotional and almost unable to do her job. When she took time out to complete a self-analysis of her reaction and the thoughts involved, here is what she came up with:

A Activating event (what started things off):
My Head of Department criticised me in front of my team.

C Consequence (how I felt and behaved):
Stayed angry all day, took it out on my team, unable to concentrate on my work.

B Beliefs (what I told myself about the A):
1 She did it because she wanted to make me look stupid in front of my team. *(mind-reading)*
2 It is horrible to be put down *(awfulising)* and I can't bear it. *(can't-stand-it-itis)*
3 She should not have done it. *(demandingness)*
4 She's a bitch. *(people-rating)*
5 I must always be treated in a fair and just manner, and it is awful and intolerable when I am not. *(core belief)*
6 People should always do the right thing. When they don't, this shows that they are bad people. *(core belief)*

E New Effect I want (how I would prefer to feel/behave):
I would prefer to feel annoyed (rather than hostile), and assertively sort it out with her (rather than brood and take it out on others).

D Disputation and new beliefs (that will help achieve the new Effect I want):

1 I have no evidence that she did it to make me look stupid in front of my team — she may have just been not thinking.

2 It is uncomfortable to be put down — not horrifying! I didn't like it, but I can (and did!) stand it.

3 It would have been better for her to have handled it differently; but where is it written that people 'should' be perfect and behave correctly at all times?

4 She is not a 'bitch' — she is just a person who sometimes does bitchy things.

5 I would prefer to always be treated fairly and justly, but nowhere is it written that I 'must'; and although I dislike poor treatment, I do survive it.

6 It would be better if people always behaved correctly — but *demanding* that reality be other than it is will only screw me up. And a bad action does not make the total person bad.

F Further action (what I will do to avoid the same self-defeating thinking and reactions in future):

1 Re-read the material on demandingness and how I can combat it.

2 Use a rational card or belief number 5 for three weeks.

3 Once every day, deliberately choose to ignore a misdemeanour on the part of my staff or other people in my life to which I would normally overreact.

How to complete a self-analysis

Here are detailed instructions for carrying out your own self-analyses. The first thing to do when you are feeling or acting in a self-defeating manner is to *stop*. Interrupt any self-defeating episodes. Take time out to get your brain working on the problem. On a good-sized sheet of paper, follow this sequence:

A Identify the Activating event

Identify and write down the stress trigger. What are you reacting to? Be brief — summarise the **A**; don't record the whole situation, just the bit you reacted to.

C Identify the Consequence

What did you feel (your emotional response), and what did you do (your behavioural response)?

B Identify your Beliefs

What were you telling yourself about the **A** that created your reaction at **C**?

1 Watch for any of the misperceptions described on page 43 — black-and-white thinking, filtering, over-generalising, mind-reading, fortune-telling, emotional reasoning, personalising.

2 Even more importantly, identify your evaluative beliefs. Look for the types described on page 40. Ask questions like:

- What am I telling myself must/should be (or not be)? *(demanding)*
- What is 'terrible'? *(awfulising)*
- What is 'unbearable'? *(can't-stand-it-itis)*
- What am I labelling myself (or others)? *(people-rating)*

3 Finally, identify the core belief(s) that are involved. Many core beliefs will be variations of the list of self-

defeating attitudes on page 44. You could use these as a prompt.

E Identify a new and better Effect

How would you prefer to feel or behave differently to your old reaction at **C**? Replace the old self-defeating reaction with more functional emotions or behaviours. Be realistic: don't attempt to replace an intense negative emotion with a strongly positive one (this would only set you up for failure); instead, substitute a more moderate negative feeling. If you are very angry, for example, do not make your goal 'to feel loving'. That would be unrealistic. It would be better to aim to be 'annoyed'. This is still a negative emotion, but more in perspective to the **A** and less disabling than hostile anger.

D Dispute and replace the old beliefs

Before you attempt to develop any new beliefs, you need to fully dispute the old ones so that you are convinced they are irrational (otherwise the new ones will not stick). To dispute a belief, ask three questions about it:

1 *Is this belief helpful or harmful?*
'Does believing this help me maintain control over myself and my life? Or does it create distress or block me from achieving my goals?'

2 *What does the evidence say?*
'What evidence is there?' 'Does it support the belief, or does the evidence really suggest some other conclusion?' 'Is there a law of Nature that proves … or is the "law" really only in my head?'

3 *Does it follow?*
'Does it logically follow that because … (I want something / it's unpleasant, I made a mistake), therefore

… (I must get what I want, it's awful, I am a total failure)?'

After disputing a belief, substitute a rational alternative. Ensure that the new belief is realistic and believable to you.

F Develop a plan for further action

Finally, consider: 'What can I do to reduce the chances of thinking and reacting the same old way in future?' There are three main types of further action, and it is usually a good idea to develop at least one item from each area:

1 *Re-education* — for example, re-reading a section of this book that is relevant to the problem you have analysed.

2 *Rethinking* — using techniques that reinforce the new beliefs (for example, *rational cards*; see page 78).

3 *Behavioural* — acting in new ways either to challenge the old beliefs by contradicting them in action, or to develop new ways of coping with problematical situations (see page 86).

Learning and using rational self-analysis

The best way to learn self-analysis is to practise it in writing. Later, you will be able to do it in your head (although at times in the future you may still find it helpful to get out pen and paper and analyse an episode more formally).

If you are like most people, you will start by doing analyses after an episode where you have already reacted. Over time, with practice, you will be able to analyse episodes while they are happening. Eventually, you will begin to anticipate self-defeating reactions and interrupt them at the start.

If you would like to learn more about the technique of rational self-analysis, it is described in more detail, along with some practice exercises, in my earlier book *Choose to be Happy*.[2]

There are many more tools that can help you deal with stress and develop a functional coping philosophy. The following sections will present a sample. Most of these techniques can be used both alone and as the 'further action' part of a rational self-analysis.

Self-education

Educate yourself about whatever it is you are trying to change. There are many sources of material (although it is important to be selective, and use material that is 'evidence-based' and that reflects a consistent approach to human problems).

Reading

Keep referring back to the sections of this book that are relevant to whatever you are working on at any given time. Acquire additional information on particular problems from other books, magazine articles, pamphlets, the Internet, and so on.

Listening

As well as reading, listening to audiotapes means you can use another of your senses to consolidate new ways of thinking. Here are some variations:

- *Pre-recorded self-help tapes*[3] have the advantage that you can listen to them while doing other things, such as housework, driving, gardening or walking.

- *Record your own tapes.* Read into your tape recorder text from books or pamphlets you find helpful and want to reuse.

- *Make tapes to help you cope with anxiety.* Record forceful rational statements, then listen to them on a portable player while carrying out anxiety-provoking behavioural assignments.

- *Tape-record a disputing sequence.* Play both the self-defeating and rational parts of yourself. Make the rational part more forceful. You could have someone else listen to your tape to check out how powerful and convincing your disputes are.

Essays

Write an essay about one of your self-defeating beliefs, debating both sides of the issue. Or research and write up in detail a particular problem area. What is known about the problem? What are the possible causes? What can be done about it? What blocks might get in the way of dealing with it? How can I overcome these blocks?

Monitoring your reactions

Diaries or *logs* are a useful way both to identify and monitor self-defeating thoughts. Keep a diary of **A**s, **B**s, and **C**s for a week or two. Use this to check out perceptions of reality (for example, 'Am I really failing all the time?'), or the extent of a problem on which you plan to work (for example, 'How often do I overeat and under what circumstances?'). Here is an example of an ABC diary:

A. Activating event	B. Beliefs/thoughts	C. Consequence
Manager criticised me in front of team.	It was horrible. She shouldn't have done it.	Angry & bitter all day.

Reinforcing new beliefs

Daily thought record

By inserting an additional **D** column, the ABC diary above becomes the 'Daily Thought Record'. This can be used as an alternative to the more detailed 'rational self-analysis' procedure described earlier.

A. Activating event	B. Beliefs/thoughts	C. Consequence	D. Disputation/ rational response
Manager criticised me in front of team.	It was horrible.	Angry & bitter all day.	It was unpleasant — not catastrophic.

Rational cards

After disputing a self-defeating belief, take a small card and write the old belief at the top and the new belief at the bottom. Carry the card with you for a week or so, and take it out of your pocket or purse and read it eight to 10 times a day. This will take less than 30 seconds each time, but the repetition can be very productive for establishing a new rational belief.

Don't be misled by the simplicity of this technique — it can be surprisingly effective. Note that a new thought requires daily practice for about three weeks before it becomes a habit, so refer to the card at least once a day for a few more weeks. Carol's card appears at the top of the next page.

Benefits calculation

This technique can be used in several different ways. It can help to break through decision-making blocks (see the example on page 320). You can also use it to increase your motivation to change, by calculating the relative advantages of change versus staying as you are (there is an example of this on page 139). To carry out a calculation, list all the

Carol's card

> **Old belief:**
>
> I must always be treated in a fair and just manner, and it is awful and intolerable when I am not.
>
> **New belief:**
>
> I would prefer to always be treated fairly and justly, but nowhere is it written that I 'must'; and though I dislike poor treatment, I do survive it.

factors that seem relevant. Determine the likelihood of short- and long-term consequences for each factor. Decide how much value or benefit each item has to you, negatively or positively, then add up the pros and cons.

Challenging demandingness

Double-standard dispute

If you are holding to a self-defeating 'should' or 'must', think of someone about whom you care very much, such as your child, partner, best friend, etc. Then consider whether you would encourage that person to hold to your demanding rule. You will almost always say an emphatic 'No!' You will then see that you are following a double standard. Ask yourself how you can justify this. (The answer will be that you can't!)

You could take this a little further, and consider what you might say to the other person to convince them of the inappropriateness of their demanding rule. You will quickly see why it is wrong for you, too. In effect, you will be arguing against your own self-defeating belief.

Carol, whose self-analysis we looked at earlier, considered whether she would want her adolescent daughter to hold her core belief that 'I must always be treated in a fair and just manner, and it is awful and intolerable when I am not.'

The answer was 'No': she did not want her own daughter to hold a belief that would lead her into a victim mentality. She rehearsed what she would say to her daughter should she ever admit to thinking in such a way — and ended up arguing quite effectively against her own self-defeating belief.

How to challenge self-rating

Double-standard dispute

The double-standard technique described above is also very useful for combating self-rating. If you are putting yourself down about something you have done or about yourself in general, think of someone who is important to you, such as a child or close friend. Then consider whether you would put *them* down for the same thing. You will almost certainly admit that you wouldn't!

When you realise that you are following a double standard which cannot be justified, it will be easier to give up the self-rating.

You could also, as with demands, go further and reflect on what you might say to the other person to talk them out of their putting themselves down — in effect, arguing against your own self-downing beliefs.

Reframing

This involves 'reframing' or viewing yourself in a different way. Instead of being, for example, 'a stupid person', you become 'a person who sometimes does stupid things'. You can do the same with all the other labels you attach to your total self: 'bad', 'selfish', 'no good', 'weak', and so on.

Be careful that you don't go to the other extreme, however, and start applying positive labels to yourself, such as 'I am a wonderful person'. This won't hold up in the long run either. Positive self-rating is just as illogical as negative self-rating — if you can be 'totally good', then you can equally well be 'totally bad'. Neither makes sense, because human beings are never one thing or the other — they are mixtures of many characteristics and tendencies. (See, also, page 58.)

Dealing with catastrophic evaluations

Catastrophe scale
Here is a technique to help you get things back into perspective when you find yourself awfulising:

1 On a sheet of paper, draw a line down one side. Put 100 per cent at the top, 0 per cent at the bottom, and fill in the rest at 10 per cent intervals.

2 Whenever you are catastrophising about something, ascertain what rating you are subconsciously giving it and pencil the item into your chart at that position.

3 Go through the other levels and at each one, write in something you think could legitimately be rated at that level. You might, for example, put:

0 per cent — 'Having a quiet cup of coffee at home';

20 per cent — 'Having to mow the lawns when the rugby is on television';

70 per cent — 'Being burgled';

90 per cent — 'Being diagnosed with cancer';

100 per cent — 'Being burned alive'; and so on.

4 Then look at how the item you are working on compares with the other items. Usually what happens is that you will realise you have been exaggerating the badness involved. Move the item down the list until you feel it is in perspective. Keep the chart and add to it from time to time. To illustrate, here is a catastrophe scale for Carol:

Carol's catastrophe scale
Issue: Being criticised in public

100	One of the children dying	original placing of issue
90	Becoming a paraplegic	
80	Being smashed up in a car accident	2nd placing
70	Being diagnosed with cancer	3rd placing
60	Husband leaving me	
50	Losing my job	
40	House burgled	
30	Losing my purse	
20	*Being criticised in public*	final placing
10	Children noisy while I watch TV	
0	Having a coffee at home	

There is another example of a catastrophe scale on page 140.

Reframing

As well as helping to combat self-rating, reframing can also be used to address catastrophising and put bad events into perspective. One way to reframe events is to re-evaluate them as 'disappointing', 'concerning' or 'uncomfortable', rather than 'awful' or 'unbearable'. Another way is to think about how even negative events almost always have a positive side to them, listing all the positives you can think of.

To ensure this technique is effective, avoid so-called 'positive' thinking and reframe only in ways that are believable to you.

Managing anxious situations

Many of the techniques already described — thought recording, rational cards, catastrophe scales and reframing — will help you manage situations about which you feel anxious. Here are some more techniques which can be used to help you manage potentially upsetting situations:

Rational-Emotive Imagery (REI)

Using the power of your imagination, REI can prepare you to deal with situations you might wish to avoid because of anxiety. Using an illustrative example, the steps are as follows:

	Procedure	Example
1	Imagine, vividly and clearly, the event or situation with which you have trouble.	You have to inform a staff member that their request for promotion has been turned down due to their poor performance record.
2	Allow yourself to feel — strongly — the self-defeating emotion that is produced by your imagining.	Anxiety.
3	Note the thoughts creating that emotion.	He will be upset. I couldn't stand feeling responsible. I must find a way to say it without him getting upset.
4	Force the emotion to change to a more functional (but realistic) feeling. It is possible to do this, even if briefly.	Concern.
5	Note the thoughts you used to change the emotion.	It will be uncomfortable, but the situation won't kill me. While I would prefer him not to get upset, his emotions are his responsibility — I cannot control his feelings or be responsible for them.
6	Practise the technique daily for a while.	

Coping rehearsal

Coping rehearsal is a variation of REI. Visualise the situation, and imagine yourself first experiencing the dysfunctional reaction, then changing your self-defeating thinking and reacting in a more func-tional way. Here are the steps:

1 Complete a rational self-analysis.

2 Imagine yourself, as vividly as you can, in the situation you are concerned about, repeating the self-defeating beliefs you listed in the analysis. Feel the emotions that follow and see yourself behaving in the self-defeating ways you anticipate.

3 Imagine yourself, still in the situation, disputing and replacing the self-defeating beliefs with the rational alternatives you developed in your analysis. Feel your negative emotion reducing to a level you can handle, and visualise yourself acting appropriately.

You can use this to prepare yourself for many situations — behaving assertively, giving a talk, coping with a job interview, negotiating a contract, and so on.

The 'blow-up' technique

Use the power of humour to put a feared situation into perspective. Imagine whatever it is you fear happening, then exaggerate it out of all proportion until you cannot help but be amused by it. Laughing at your fears will help you get control of them.

Carol, for example, was afraid to be assertive with a colleague, Joe, who frequently dumped his work onto her. She visualised telling Joe how she felt when it happened. She 'saw' Joe accusing her loudly of being selfish and unwilling to work as part of a team, the rest of the office gathering around and agreeing with him, management called in to deal with her, the police summoned to take her away, her picture and a description of her actions broadcast on the television news, the country in uproar, the government passing an Act to have her personally restrained from ever confronting anyone again, and the army, complete with tanks and artillery, patrolling her workplace to make sure she stayed in line.

Time projection

This technique is designed to show that one's life, and the world in general, will continue after a feared or unwanted event has come and gone.

Visualise the event occurring, then imagine going forwards in time a week, then a month, then six months; then a year, two years, and so on. Consider how you are likely to be feeling at each of these points in time. You will eventually see that life will go on, even though you may need to make some adjustments.

You can use this with a range of events and circumstances, such as actual or feared redundancy, loss of a contract, business failure, reduction in income, death of a loved one, disability, failure to pass an examination, and so on.

The worry calculator

This technique is a quick way to put worrying into perspective. Draw four boxes as shown overleaf. List everthing about which you typically worry, or are worrying over at the present time. To ensure that no significant items are missed, you could keep a 'worry diary' for a week or so. Areas to look at may include *personal* health, well-being, comfort, success and safety; *family* health, finances and children's welfare; *job-related* concerns, performance and people; *global* issues, war and disasters; and the *little things* to which you react.

	Things I can do something about	Things I can't do anything about
Important to me	I	II
Not important to me	IV	III

Be realistic about which box you place an item in. Don't put impossible items (for example, to 'always avoid disapproval') in Boxes I or IV, or things about which you could do something (for example, getting behind with tasks) in Boxes II or III. Also, make realistic decisions as to what is important and what is not.

Finally, develop some strategies to problem-solve on the items in Box I (see Chapter 19); and work at acceptance (see page 119) for the items in Box II.

Developing new behaviours

It is important to put your cognitive changes into actual practice. Behavioural techniques, or 'action assignments', will help you in a number of ways. You can deepen and consolidate rational beliefs by acting in accordance with the new beliefs and in opposition to the old, self-defeating ones. You can raise your tolerance for frustration and discomfort by deliberately exposing yourself to these. And you can experiment with and practise new ways of handling problematical situations.

Exposure

Exposure involves deliberately putting yourself into real-life situations you might otherwise avoid. There are three main purposes: (1) to test out the accuracy or otherwise of beliefs (like, for example, that you can't stand rejection, by actually risking it); (2) to increase tolerance for discomfort; and (3) to practise new ways of dealing with situations. Exposure can be a powerful tool for increasing control over yourself and your life.

It is helpful to deliberately set up the situations rather than wait for them to occur. This allows you to prepare for them, so they are under your control. Practising in this planned and managed way will then help you cope when events happen unexpectedly. Here are some of the ways you can use exposure:

- *Shame-attacking* involves doing things you have previously avoided through fear of what other people might think. It will increase your tolerance for discomfort, reduce your concern about disapproval, and increase your ability to take (sensible) risks. The actions need to be such that other people are likely to notice and disapprove of them. For example:

  —If you are obsessive about your appearance, leave home wearing unmatched items of clothing or without your usual grooming.

  —If you worry about behaving correctly in front of others, break some minor social convention.

  —Face any fear of being seen as stupid by expressing an opinion to a group of people.

- *Risk-taking* will help you challenge beliefs that certain behaviours are too dangerous to risk, when reason tells you that, while the outcome is not guaranteed, they are worth the chance. For example:

—Combat perfectionism or fear of failure by starting tasks where there is a good chance of failing or not matching your expectations.

—Face fear of rejection by seeking it out — for example, talk to an attractive person at a party, or ask someone to go out with you.

- *Desensitisation* involves deliberately entering situations you fear in order to demonstrate to yourself that you can at least survive them, if not learn to handle them. For example, if you are afraid of being in lifts, go into a lift several times a day until the fear diminishes.

There is an example of exposure applied to the management of anger on page 143. If you would like to learn more about exposure, it is discussed in detail in my book on anxiety management, *FearLess*.[4]

Paradoxical behaviour

When you have difficulty with things like perfectionism or handling frustration, deliberately act in a way that contradicts the old tendency. Behaving in new ways will help you change such tendencies. Here are some examples:

- *Step out of character.* If you have perfectionist tendencies, deliberately do some tasks to less than your usual standard. If you feel guilty because you think you are a 'selfish' person, treat yourself in some way each day for a week. If you tend to rush round a lot but worry you are not getting enough done, deliberately slow down and take long breaks where you do nothing but relax.

- *Postpone gratification.* If your problem is undue frustration when you have to wait for what you want, deliberately delay gratification with something each day for a month or two.

Role-playing

Role-playing difficult situations will enable you to test out and practise different ways of coping with them before you face the real thing. Role-playing is often used when a situation involves communicating with others. Practising assertiveness is a common example.

Role-play with a trusted friend or colleague. Repeat the role-play until you feel you have got it right. Get the other person to give you feedback on how you came across so that you can gradually refine your technique.

Some notes on using behavioural techniques

Before commencing exposure, prepare yourself in advance with *imagery* (page 83), where you go through the exposure in your imagination before using it in real life. Depending on what you are confronting, *role-playing* as described above may give you confidence. Completing a *benefits calculation* (page 78) will aid your motivation by clarifying the gains you will achieve. Prior to entering the exposure situation, and when you are in it, use a *rational card* (page 78) to refresh your recollection of helpful new ways of thinking. If you become tense, use a relaxation technique (see Chapter 10).

Don't take foolhardy risks. Avoid doing anything that might cause injury, or unduly alarm or disrupt the lives of others.

Keep in mind that the object of action assignments is not to 'succeed'. The real purpose is to expose yourself to problematical situations, either to test them out or increase your tolerance. If your risk-taking always succeeded, you would do little to raise your tolerance for discomfort. Often what you fear will not actually occur — but it is better that it sometimes does. For example, you are more likely to be confident that you could handle rejection when you have actually been rejected a few times.

You can either start at the deep end and tackle the things that bother you most, or take a graduated approach. With the latter, start by preparing a list of the things you find difficult, and order them into a hierarchy according to the level of anxiety you associate with each one. Then confront the situations systematically, working your way up from the low-anxiety items through to the high-level ones. Don't try to avoid all discomfort. If you make it too easy, you will do little to increase your tolerance. Develop assignments that are 'challenging but not overwhelming'. Again, you can prepare yourself in advance of confronting a problematical situation by using the techniques described earlier: imagery can help you cope emotionally; role-playing can give you confidence.

And remember: for new behaviours to consolidate, you will usually need to carry them out on a number of occasions over a period of time.

Making Rational Effectiveness Training work for you

The techniques you have learned from this chapter will be very helpful as you seek to manage yourself and your life more effectively. But they will only work if you actually use them — and keep on using them. Bear in mind, too, that even though you may have been coping well for a while, human beings tend to revert back to previous self-defeating methods of coping when under pressure. It is important, therefore, not to become discouraged when you find yourself worrying again or avoiding discomfort like you did in the past. Use this as a signal that you are under extra stress, and need to dust off the coping skills you have learned and once again put them into practice.

As time goes on, the new ways of reacting will become more automatic, especially if you use slip-backs as further opportunities to practise your coping skills, rather than see them as events that 'shouldn't' happen. Look on them as inevitable short-term experiences that you can use to your long-term advantage.

7

Worrying:
when your brain has a mind of its own

Author's note: Worrying is covered extensively in *FearLess*,[1] my book on anxiety management. However, because it is highly relevant to the issues of stress and control, especially over the mind, a summarised and slightly modified form of the material from *FearLess* is reproduced here.

It is wise to be concerned about the chance of things going wrong in your life. Concern can keep you alert and motivate you to fix them. Unfortunately for some people, however, concern gets out of hand. They think obsessively about their problems but do little to solve them. Or they just feel anxious about 'everything'. For them, concern has turned into 'worry'.

People can worry about almost anything. The most common fears involve finances, work performance, social coping, or the possibility of an illness or accident. For some, the symptoms can cause significant distress and difficulties with work, social or personal functioning.

Most people who worry would rather not. Unfortunately, however, it is hard to stop the flow of unwanted thoughts. People even worry about not worrying, fearing that bad things will creep up if they are not constantly on the alert.

In this chapter, you will learn why human beings worry, why you don't need to, and what you can do to take control over a mind that seems to have a mind of its own.

To illustrate this problem, let's meet Paul, a 46-year-old self-employed builder. His business was successful and his home life stable — but this didn't stop him worrying. He had worried since childhood, the tendency worsening as he got older. His typical worries were about money, the security of his business, the health of his wife and children, whether he would still have friends in the future, anything that might potentially go wrong with his car, work that needed doing on his house . . . In fact, just about anything he put his mind to was a potential subject for apprehension.

The worrying created stomach pains and cost him sleep, his productivity was declining because he worried instead of doing, and his wife was tired of constantly hearing about what might go wrong in the future. Unfortunately, Paul found it next to impossible to control his worrying thoughts.

What is worrying?

Worry refers to a chain or stream of negative thoughts and images about concerns, usually related to the future. It involves a combination of *obsessive thinking* about how to solve or avoid problems, and *catastrophising* about the possible consequences of those problems. Put another way, you are worrying when you obsessively think about your problems, and fear what they might lead to, but do little about them. Worrying is a way of *thinking*. It leads to the set of *feelings* we call *anxiety*: tension, apprehensiveness, frustration, upset stomach, and so on.

Anxiety is a normal 'warning bell'. The feelings are designed to alert us to possible danger and, ideally, to motivate us to take action to deal with the danger. Worrying, however, while *seemingly* aimed at finding solutions to problems, usually has the opposite result. When people worry, they foresee bad things happening and feel anxious; but instead of doing anything about their worries, they just keep 'ruminating' — mulling the worries over and over in their minds. Whereas *appropriate anxiety* leads to action — after which the symptoms subside — *worry* just goes on and on.

This was Denise's experience. A hard-working mother of two, Denise worked as a receptionist-typist for a large medical practice. Her husband Nigel was a senior manager with a software manufacturer. Denise was thinking about a message from Joan, her practice manager, that signalled some changes to Denise's conditions of employment. Denise was not happy with the changes. But instead of clarifying what she did want, Denise just kept mulling over what might happen if she disagreed with Joan, feeling increasingly tense and upset.

Why do people worry?

Worry originates with the natural (and quite rational) human tendency to reflect on problems and dangers in order to solve or avoid them. But, like many other human tendencies, this natural concern can become exaggerated and take on a life of its own — causing a person to keep thinking about a problem but do nothing to deal with it.

Possibly the main reason why many people keep worrying is this: *they think it somehow protects them from danger*. Underlying this are beliefs like: 'I must always be prepared for danger'; 'If I don't worry, bad things might creep up on me'; or 'If I worry, I can stop bad things happening'.

Worry also becomes a *habit*, which makes it hard to

stop. Believing that worry 'stops bad things happening' gets reinforced because, usually, nothing does happen — which leads the worrier to assume, superstitiously, that this was because they worried!

Emotional reasoning plays a part — thinking that because you *feel* anxious, this somehow *proves* that something bad is likely to happen. By creating fearful images in the mind, worrying feeds the idea that danger really does exist.

Worrying is often fuelled by *demands for safety* — that life must be completely safe; certain things must be guaranteed; one's marriage, home, money, job, etc must be totally protected. If you view anything as an absolute *need* rather than as a *preference*, then you are likely to worry about it. And if you believe that 'there *must* be a perfect solution to every problem', then whenever you are faced by a situation that does not have an obvious 'best' choice, you are likely to put off doing anything.

Self-image issues may be involved. Some people think it is 'caring' or 'responsible' to worry, believing 'If I didn't worry, that would show I was an uncaring/irresponsible person.' And a person who is overly concerned about disapproval or criticism from other people will tend to worry about making mistakes, looking foolish, or saying or doing the 'wrong' thing. Similarly, someone who lacks confidence in their ability to cope with life's demands and stresses will be more likely to worry about the chance of them happening.

For Denise, worry had been a lifetime habit. She often felt uncomfortable when she was not worrying, believing that worry somehow protected her from danger creeping up and catching her unawares. Underlying this tendency were internal demands, self-taught in childhood, that 'life must be safe' and that 'I must ensure that nothing bad happens to me or my family unless I am prepared for it.' She also believed that she would be an irresponsible person if she did not worry about the possibility of danger to her family.

The vicious circle of worrying

Worrying involves a vicious circle. An activating event triggers the core beliefs that predispose you to worry. This creates symptoms of anxiety. You interpret the symptoms as a warning of danger. This increases the anxiety. A loop is thus set up — focussing on the worrying and the symptoms effectively takes your attention away from the original problem.

What you can do about it

Now let's move on from the problem to the solution. The aims of a programme to take control over worrying, along with strategies for achieving these aims, are as follows:

- to *restrain obsessive worrying*, using rational thinking and problem-solving techniques
- to *control physical symptoms* with relaxation and breathing control
- to *reduce avoidance behaviour* by using graduated exposure
- to *solve life problems* more effectively using new skills
- to *develop a lifestyle that minimises worrying*, by changing self-defeating behaviours.

Start by clarifying the problem

Is the worrying a feature of your life in general — or has it begun recently or does it occur only under certain circumstances? In the latter case, there may be other issues to check out. Depression (page 25) can cause an increase in worrying. If you are experiencing anxiety resulting from trauma, see page 23 for advice on this. Consult your doctor if you have a general medical disorder like, for example, hyperthyroidism or diabetes.

Be aware of any substances that may be inducing anxiety, for example, excessive caffeine, some medications, various illegal drugs, etc. You will need to do something about the substance use before anything else; consult your health advisor. Think about whether there are any other lifestyle factors that may contribute to worrying, such as inadequate exercise.

Log your worrying patterns

When you are ready to begin work on the worrying itself, the first step is to make a list of your symptoms and behaviour patterns. The best way to do this is by keeping a log for two to four weeks. Here are the items to record:

- *What do you typically worry about?*
  This might include such things as dealing with financial matters; tackling tasks about which you lack confidence; acting assertively with others; you or a loved one becoming ill; making mistakes; upsetting others; and so on.

- *What do you typically avoid?*
  Watch for procrastination, delaying decisions, neglecting everyday tasks (such as paying bills), or failing to check out concerns (such as not going to the doctor to get a lump checked). This will provide additional clues as to what you worry about. Avoidance of balancing the cheque book or paying bills may reflect worrying about money; putting things off at work may suggest that you are worrying about your performance.

- *What do you experience while you are worrying?*
  Do you experience muscular tension, raised heartbeat, headaches? Do you have panic attacks (see page 24)? Is your concentration poor? Are you restless? Is it hard to settle to tasks? Are you having trouble sleeping? Recording the symptoms will enable you to address them more directly.

Develop your plan

When you have clarified the specific problems you are having with worrying, turn these problems into goals and develop a self-help plan.

Clarify your goals

List the goals for your self-help plan. As far as possible, state them in specific, behavioural terms, like, for example:

- 'Reduce my episodes of worry to 30 minutes maximum'

- 'Know how to problem-solve difficult issues'

- 'Balance my cheque book within one week of receiving the monthly bank statement'

- 'Wean myself off tranquillisers'.

Aim to minimise your worrying as far as possible, but not to eliminate it entirely — otherwise you will set yourself up to be disillusioned. Striving for management rather than cure will almost certainly increase your chances of success.

Set up your self-help plan

Next, develop a plan to achieve the goals you have set. This will be based on the information you collected during the clarifying phase. List the various strategies and techniques you will use to achieve your self-help goals. These might include any of the following:

- self-education about the nature of worrying and anxiety in general

- re-thinking strategies to reduce worrying (for example, reality-checking, stimulus control) — the 'six-step worry plan', which we shall discuss shortly, is possibly the most effective strategy here

- relaxation training or breathing control to reduce tension and other physical symptoms

- exposure to any activities and situations you have been avoiding

- changing any dysfunctional core beliefs

- learning to use problem-solving or assertiveness training to deal with issues that do need attention

- lifestyle changes where appropriate.

The basics of overcoming worry

Before you put your self-help plan into action, it will help to understand some facts about worry. Probably the most important fact is that worrying, as we have defined it in this chapter, is not as important to your survival as you might have believed.

Accept that worrying is not helpful

Worrying has *no* positive benefits. It does not help you avoid danger or solve problems. In fact, it gets in the way of problem-solving! It is unproductive, leading to procrastination rather than action. It affects the body, creating stomach ulcers, muscular tension and headaches.

It stops people enjoying the present moment by keeping them focussed on what might happen in the future. And the longer you worry about something, the worse it seems.

Remember: worrying does not ward off danger. Bad things happen to good people, no matter how much they worry. Worrying just adds further emotional pain on top of the bad events that do occur in your life. So, the first step is to remind yourself that worrying is both bad for you and unnecessary. Completing the *worry calculator* on page 85 would be a good way to begin getting your worrying in perspective.

Have a replacement for worry

Simply telling yourself to 'stop worrying' is usually not enough, because sometimes there are things which do require attention.

. What you need is a realistic replacement for worry. The best alternative is to be 'concerned'. How does concern differ from worry? It is still a negative emotion — but it is not as draining, and it leads to action rather than rumination. Make concern your aim.

Have a process to use when you find yourself worrying

Finally, have some kind of procedure you can follow when you realise that you have slipped into worrying again, such as the 'six-step worry plan'.

The six-step worry plan

Worrying is a hard habit to break. The six-step plan provides a well-structured procedure you can use to beat it. Here is a summary of what is involved:

1 *Catch yourself worrying, then pause.* To combat worrying, you need to recognise when you are doing it.

2 *Identify the real issue.* Find out what it is you are really concerned about.

3 *Do a reality check.* Ask yourself: 'How likely is it that what I fear will happen?' and 'How bad would it be if it did occur?'

4 *Decide whether action is required.* 'Do I need to do anything about this — or is it something that is unlikely to happen (or about which nothing can be done anyway)?'

5 When the thing you fear *is* likely to be a reality, then *get into action* to problem-solve it.

6 If, on the other hand, you decide that the worry is not really an issue, then use some psychological strategies to *let it go*.

Let's look at these steps in greater detail.

Step 1. Pause

Catch yourself doing it

Pick up on the early signs of worrying. Worrying, and its attendant anxiety, is much easier to inhibit at an early stage before it begins to spiral. Learn to monitor yourself. Note any signs that indicate you may be starting to worry:

- You feel uncomfortable, anxious, tense or unhappy.
- You are mulling something over but doing little about it.
- You are predicting catastrophic consequences.
- You are avoiding tackling something that you find uncomfortable.

Also note whatever triggers these responses. Acknowledge

that you are worrying instead of problem-solving; and that this not only feels bad but is unproductive. *Stop drifting* — consciously stop, and *take action*. You might find it helpful to keep a diary for a few weeks to help identify the signs to watch for.

Denise eventually realised that her tension, upset stomach and poor concentration meant that she was worrying again, so she decided to sit down with pen and paper to analyse what was going on in her mind.

Make an initial decision on what to do with the worry

With some worries, it will be helpful to go through all of the steps that remain; for others, you can skip some steps and deal more quickly with the issue:

- If you are already clear in your mind as to what you are really worried about, skip straight to step 3.

- If you think the issue is not worth worrying about at all, go straight to step 6.

- If it seems like the issue is important, but you don't have time to deal with it immediately, make a commitment to get back to it at a certain time — and let go of the worry for the interim. If letting go is difficult, see the strategies under step 6.

Step 2. Identify your real concerns

Sometimes you will be quite clear in your mind as to what the real issue is. In such cases you can proceed straight to step 3.

At other times, however, you will be aware only of vague feelings of discomfort, or you will have identified the trigger to your worries but not the underlying issue.

List your concerns and select the main one

Start by asking yourself questions like: 'What am I bothered about?' or 'What is the issue?' Write down the answers. You may well have more than one thing on your mind, but just focus on listing the worries.

If this is difficult because the worrying seems to be unfocussed, it may be helpful to pause, sit down, allow yourself to be aware of the feelings of discomfort in your body, and focus your mind on them. Then ask the questions again.

Denise listed four things that were on her mind to some degree:

1 The message from Joan.

2 Her son Liam had complained of toothache before school that morning.

3 She had received a larger-than-usual electricity bill a week earlier.

4 Nigel had begun talking about leaving his secure job and setting up a business of his own.

If there is more than one item on your list, as there often will be, ask yourself: 'Which of these things am I most worried about? Which is contributing most to my feelings of discomfort?' You will usually make this choice intuitively (re-focussing on the physical sensations of discomfort may help you do this). Whichever thought you choose becomes what we will call the 'key issue' or 'key concern'.

Denise relaxed herself, cleared her mind and concentrated on the feeling of anxiety. Before long, an image of her manager sitting at her desk floated into her mind. She deduced from this that the issue with Joan was the key concern on which to work.

Collect thoughts about the key concern

What are you telling yourself about the key issue? What is it you are most bothered about? At this stage just 'collect' thoughts, like you did when you were listing the concerns; except this time you are looking for the *thoughts* you have about your key concern.

Denise listed three thoughts:

1 The changes could mean less flexibility in my hours.

2 If I don't say anything I will feel resentful.

3 If I disagree with Joan, she will think I am being difficult.

Choose the key thought

The next step is to choose the 'key thought' — the one that you intuitively sense is most associated with the anxious feeling. Denise decided that her key thought was: 'If I disagree with Joan, she will think I am being difficult.'

Follow the chain from the key thought

Now expand on the key thought in order to identify the main underlying issue. You are seeking to answer questions like the following: 'What, ultimately, am I anxious about? What exactly am I predicting will happen, and what is the crucial issue with that?'

You achieve this by using a process known as 'chaining'. Worrying thoughts usually run in chains, with one link of the chain leading to another; like, for example:

'If Nigel goes into business we will be even more short of money for a long time.' → 'We will have to cut back.' → 'The kids will go without.' → 'My mother will criticise me for not caring for them properly.' → 'I would feel bad about myself.'; and so on.

Move down the chain, asking yourself questions like: 'What really bothers me about that?' or 'What is worrying about that?' or 'If that were true, what would it mean to me?' and so on. Denise began the chaining process by asking herself:

1 *Assuming it is true that Joan will think I am being difficult, what would that mean to me?* The answer was: 'She will think less of me.'

2 *And if she thinks less of me?* Denise came up with two replies here: (1) 'She will be less keen to help me develop my career' and (2) 'She will tell other people I am difficult.' Denise then considered which was the new 'key thought', and chose option (1).

3 *If she was less keen to help my career, what would bother me about that?* 'My career will suffer, I will not advance.'

4 *And if my career did not advance, what is worrying about that for me?* 'My mother will think I'm a failure.'

5 *And if she thought I was a failure, what would that mean to me?* 'I couldn't stand that, it would be unbearable.'

Identify your evaluation-thinking

Note that in the above example, Denise is engaged in two types of worrying thinking. First, most of her thoughts are perceptions or inferences (statements about what she thinks will actually happen) — for example, 'My mother will think I'm a failure.'

Second, she evaluates her inferences (for example, '… it would be *unbearable*'). It is usually the evaluative thoughts that create distress, and most thinking chains end with them. As we saw earlier in the book, there are four main types of evaluative thinking that cause trouble for human beings:

- *Demanding* — putting 'shoulds' and 'musts' on yourself (and perhaps onto others). Ask: 'What demands are involved? What am I telling myself *should* or *must* be; or *should not* or *must not* happen?' 'Am I thinking I *must* worry, otherwise (a) something bad will happen or (b) it would mean I was "uncaring"?'

- *Awfulising* — evaluating something as horrible, terrible or the worst thing that could happen. Ask: 'What am I thinking would be awful/terrible/horrible?'

- *Can't-stand-it-itis* — viewing something as 'unbearable' or 'intolerable'. Ask: 'What threat to my comfort do I fear?' 'What would be "unbearable" if it occurred?'

- *Self-rating* — evaluating your total self on the basis of one or a few characteristics or behaviours. Ask: 'What threat to my self-image do I fear?' 'What do I think such and such would "prove" about *me as a person* if it were to happen?'

What kind of evaluative thinking was Denise engaging in? She identified *can't-stand-it-itis* ('... it would be unbearable'). She realised she was evaluating her mother's criticism as 'unbearable' because she subconsciously believed that if she were to *fail at something important* this would somehow prove she was a *failure as a person*. On further reflection, she realised that underlying this was a demand: 'To be OK as a person I *must* achieve and succeed at whatever I do, and never fail at anything that is important to me.' This represents a 'core belief' (see page 42).

Step 2 may seem rather laborious at first glance, but it is worth the time and effort. Face it — you are already using up a lot of time and energy by worrying! Time spent combating it now will save a lot of time in the future.

Step 3. Do a reality check on your concerns

Having identified your real concerns, now it's time to check them out. Use the three disputational questions introduced in the previous chapter (page 74) to check out each worrying thought:

1 'How does this thought affect me?'

2 'What's the evidence?' and

3 'Does my conclusion follow from the evidence?'

How does this thought affect me?

'Is it helpful or harmful to believe this?' Ask this question about any type of worrying thought. Consider: what are the benefits and the costs of worrying versus the benefits and costs of being concerned?

Denise decided that her underlying demand to succeed actually blocked her from getting on with things where success was not guaranteed; and, additionally, created unnecessary anguish and anxiety.

What does the evidence say?

'What is the evidence both for and against believing that x will occur, or that it will occur in the way I predict?' This question is mainly relevant to inferential-type thoughts, or perceptions. Some specific things to consider are:

- 'What is (a) the worst that could happen; (b) the best that could happen; and (c) the most likely to happen?'

- 'What are the chances (on a 0–100 per cent scale) that these things will actually occur; and the chances that they won't?'

- 'What does the evidence suggest?'

- 'How often in the past have my worries actually happened — and how often have they not?'

Denise realised that her chain of inferences about what her boss Joan would think was not supported by the evidence. In fact, past experience showed that Joan usually listened and took a reasonable position with her staff when they disagreed with her. Denise did consider it likely, however, that if her career did ever suffer for some reason, her mother probably *would* criticise her — but challenged the idea that her mother's views somehow proved something about her.

Does it follow?

'Does if logically follow that if x happened, therefore y would be the case?' This question is particularly useful with evaluative thoughts.

Denise challenged her underlying demand that she 'must' succeed, asking herself: 'Does it logically follow that because it would be *desirable* to achieve, that therefore I *absolutely must*? And how does it follow that when I fail at something I go from being OK as a person to not-OK?' The answer, of course, is that neither of these follows.

Summary of the disputation process

There is more information about disputing self-defeating beliefs on page 74. To summarise, here are the questions to consider:

- 'What is the *evidence*?' 'What is the likelihood that what I fear will actually happen?'

- 'Where is it written that because I *prefer* bad things not to happen, therefore they *must* not happen?'

- 'If it did happen, would it really be awful or *unbearable* — or rather *unpleasant* but survivable?'

- 'Would such and such an event really prove something about the *kind of person* I am?'

Step 4. Decide what to do

The next step is to decide what to do about the issue of concern:

- Does the issue need attention? If so, either get on to it immediately, or make a concrete plan to attend to it later. Be very specific about what actions you will take and when you will take them. (See step 5.)

- If you decide the issue is not really important after all, then let it go. If you find letting go difficult, as most people who worry do, see the strategies described in step 6.

Step 5. Problem-solve when necessary

For issues that really do require some action, structured problem-solving will help you plan such action. Follow these steps:

1 Collect information. What are the facts?

2 Clarify exactly what the problem is.

3 Identify the causes.

4 List all the options for action that are available.

5 Decide on the most likely options.

6 Carry out the actions you have decided on.

Ask: 'Can I sort this out myself, or would I be better to obtain some help? If the latter, who can I ask, and what is stopping me from doing this?' See Chapter 19 for more detailed instructions on problem-solving.

Step 6. Let go of a persistent worry

What do you do when you have checked out a worry and either problem-solved it or decided it does not need attention, but you still can't get it out of your mind? The answer is to apply strategies that will help you let it go.

Break the connection between your worry and its triggers

If the conditions under which worrying happens are restricted, then it gradually becomes associated with fewer and fewer triggers or 'stimuli'. With this in mind, Thomas Borkovec and his associates at Pennsylvania State University developed a technique known as 'stimulus control'. It involves interrupting worry whenever it is triggered off, 'postponing' it until a set time each day. The idea of postponing worry may sound a bit strange at first, but people find it surprisingly effective once they try it. Postponing breaks the connection between a worry and its trigger. The procedure is as follows:

1 Schedule a 15–30 minute 'worry period' for the same time each day (the evening is usually best).

2 Postpone all worrying until that set time. Tell yourself you will focus on the issue later. (Do the same if you wake in the night and find yourself worrying.) To help get the worry out of your mind in the meantime, write it down in a notebook (carry this around with you, and keep it by your bedside).

   You might also find it helpful to use distraction techniques (discussed shortly), or work out the anxiety with physical exercise — walking, jogging, swimming, etc.

3 When you come to the worry period, go through the concerns you have postponed and decide which of them are still issues (many will not be). Use problem-solving on the ones that you decide *do* need action, and let go of the others.

Distract your mind

Once you have decided that a particular worry is not justified, you can inhibit the obsessive thinking by distracting yourself in numerous ways. Here are some examples:

- Entertainment: watching TV, listening to music.

- Physical activity: gardening, home maintenance, household tasks, walking, jogging, swimming, etc.

- Absorbing activities: using a computer, reading, arts and crafts, doing a puzzle.

- Relaxation: one useful approach that can be learned quickly is the 'breathing-focus' technique described on page 181. This method not only relaxes the body but also clears the mind.

Begin by making your own list of suitable distractions. Keep the list where you know you can find it when you are worrying. (However, don't use distraction to put off problem-solving when there is something that really does need attention. Such avoidance may only lead to more serious worrying later on.)

Interrupt the worrying

There is a technique called 'thought-stopping' that you can use to cut short an episode of obsessive worrying. Like distraction, thought-stopping will help only temporarily, but it can be useful to break obsessive patterns of thinking. The basic strategy is to stop an unwanted thought or image by interrupting it. There are three ways to achieve this — which is best for you will depend on whether you prefer to hear things, see them or feel them. Here is the procedure for the 'auditory' person:

1 Hold the obsessive thought in your mind for about 10 seconds, then shout 'Stop!' in a loud voice.

2 Repeat this 10–20 times, until you become used to it.

3 Practise for a few days at home or in other situations where you can shout without others noticing.

4 When you are ready, begin to shout 'Stop!' subvocally (that is, in your mind). From this point on you will be able use thought-stopping wherever you happen to be when anxious thoughts intrude.

If you are more 'visual', try the *traffic light approach*. When you have the unwanted thought, visualise a picture of a big traffic light in your mind, with the red light coming on.

For the 'feeling' person, the *rubber band technique* may work best. Place a rubber band around one of your wrists. Whenever you have the unwanted thought, flick the rubber band just hard enough for it to sting. The pain serves to interrupt the obsessive thought.

A further alternative approach is to *focus on the environment*. Instead of saying 'stop', visualising a red light or flicking a rubber band, concentrate on your current surroundings and describe (aloud when possible) its various aspects in painstaking detail.

You can use *alternative imagery* to enhance thought-stopping: after inhibiting the anxious thought or image, substitute a coping thought or pleasant fantasy.

Keep in mind that thought-stopping will appear attractive because it can be quickly learned and involves little discomfort, but it may be a way of simply avoiding uncomfortable thoughts. Thought-stopping, therefore, is best used when self-defeating beliefs have been fully analysed, and you just need to combat some remaining habitual thoughts.

Use rational cards

On a small pocket-sized card, write down the key *worrying* thought followed by a *rational alternative* thought as a counter. Carry the card with you and read it 8–10 times daily until the worry diminishes. Then keep the card handy to re-read whenever the worrying thoughts return. See page 78 for more on using this simple but effective technique.

Release your tension

Learn how to reduce the tension in your body. Two ways to do this are the *breathing-focus technique* (page 181) and *progressive relaxation training* (page 169). Relaxation can be very helpful when tension makes it hard to get to sleep, as well as generally reducing the 'alarm signals' that your tense body is sending to your mind. The breathing-focus technique is an excellent way to clear the mind as well as relax the body.

Project your worry into the future

Time projection (see page 85) is a simple yet effective technique to combat catastrophising and get a feared event into perspective.

- Visualise the unwanted event occurring, then imagine going forward in time two days, then a week, then a month, then six months, then a year, two years, and so on.

- As you come to each point of time in your imagination, consider how you will be feeling at that point.

What usually happens is that people envisage feeling better the further in time they get from the event. Time projection will help you see that if a bad event did occur, life would go on, even though you might need to make some adjustments.

Talk it over

Talking through a worry with someone else can help sort fact from fiction, and can aid problem-solving. Even just verbalising a concern to someone who does little else but listen can help reduce the pressure. If necessary, explain to your helpers that what you want is for them to mainly listen — not to judge, interrupt, or give advice except when you request it.

Putting it all together

Denise, whose worrying tendency was a lifetime problem, decided that stimulus control would be a useful technique to develop. She set aside 7.00–7.30 p.m. as her 'worry period'. Whenever she found herself worrying rather than acting, she wrote down the worry item in a notebook she kept with her. Then, if the worrying thought intruded again, she combated it with a technique appropriate for the situation she was in at the time. At work, she read a rational card and then occupied herself with an absorbing task. Walking home, she distracted herself from worrying thoughts by closely observing the views around her. At home, she used the breathing-focus technique. She some-times used thought-stopping for especially intrusive thoughts. At 7.00 p.m. she opened up her notebook and looked through her worry list. Many items seemed unimportant by then and she simply crossed them off. If an item merited attention, she analysed it in more detail, using problem-solving where appropriate. As time went by, she found she needed to record items in her notebook less and less, because her brain began to internalise the message that worrying served no useful purpose.

Dealing with a resistant worry

When a worry seems especially difficult to deal with, ask yourself three questions:

1 'What is it about this worry that makes it hard to let go?'
   —What are the possibilities? (Brainstorm ideas.)
   —What is the worst that could happen? What do I really fear?
   —Am I afraid that the consequences will reflect on my self-image, or affect how I live my life, or both?
   —What could there be that might actually need attending to? Or is my concern exaggerated?
   —Is there some reason why I might be hanging on to it? Am I afraid of what will happen if I act?

2 'What is the outcome I would really prefer to see?'
   —How would I like to see this concern resolved?

3 'What strategies and techniques could I be using here?'
   —What have I tried that hasn't worked? Why might it have failed?
   —What haven't I tried yet? Why not?
   —Have I done a rational self-analysis on this worry? Would it be helpful to do one?
   —Could I be using stimulus control or distraction or some other technique?

—Would it help to talk it over with someone? Who could I talk with?

—What could I do right now to ease the worry?

Confront what you fear

The more you avoid situations you fear, the more they build up in your mind. Conversely, if you repeatedly face your fears, you will discover that they rarely come to pass. As a result, over time you will 'extinguish' your unrealistic fears. 'Real-life exposure' (page 87) is a crucial part of overcoming anxiety. It is usually most effective to face feared situations in a graduated way, and only after you have developed rethinking skills, relaxation, and other coping strategies you can use while in the exposure situation.

Identify your avoidance

Start by preparing two lists. In the first, identify any 'big' things you have been avoiding, such as going to the doctor to have something checked, tackling a contentious issue with another person, seeing an accountant about your debts, starting an academic assignment, and so on. These may have accumulated if you have been worrying more than usual.

In the second list, write down the things that you typically avoid in your everyday life. These may be harder to identify because they are more routine. Procrastination is a common avoidance behaviour: look for tendencies such as putting bills aside, delaying decisions, neglecting to balance your cheque book, putting off tasks for which you lack confidence, failing to act assertively with other people. It will probably help to keep a log (page 77) for a while to identify these subtle types of avoidance behaviour.

Major avoidance: carry out graduated exposure

For the 'big' items on your first list, select several items with which to begin, develop exposure hierarchies for each, and get started on the first step. Re-read the material on exposure (page 87) for instructions on setting up and carrying out exposure hierarchies.

Routine avoidance: act or plan

Tackle the items on your second list by either acting on them immediately, or putting them aside with a definite arrangement to take action on them at a specific time. With the latter approach, be on the alert for two unhelpful outcomes: you continue to worry or — at the other extreme —you simply forget to deal with the issue at all.

If you find yourself continuing to worry, repeat steps 3 and 4 of the six-step plan. If the issue needs attention now rather than later, proceed with step 5.

If important issues are being forgotten, reflect on why that may be happening. One possibility is that you need to develop a more efficient reminder system. Or you might be so anxious about the issue that you are suppressing the anxiety and subconsciously 'forgetting' as a way to avoid dealing with it. If the latter, make yourself confront the issue. You could do this by completing a full rational self-analysis (page 70) and then, if necessary, doing some exposure work to tackle it directly.

Beyond letting go

Analysing a worry and letting it go is only part of the picture. There are some other things you can do to decrease your worrying tendency in the long term.

Take preventative action

As you start to get a grip on your worry, begin developing

strategies that will reduce the likelihood of it happening in the first place.

Could you make some changes to your lifestyle? Do you worry about such things as overspending, indebtedness, your health, job, and the like? Are there lifestyle factors that increase your feelings of anxiety: overusing stimulants such as sugar or caffeine, insufficient exercise, or substance abuse? If so, make a list of these factors. Keep a diary for a month or two of all the things you worry about, then summarise the themes that emerge. Use problem-solving (see Chapter 19) to help make changes.

Plan ahead. Identify the things you typically worry about, then develop strategies to handle those situations more effectively. For example, if you worry about being on time, you might get a second alarm clock to wake you in the morning, or a digital organiser to remind you of appointments. Plan in advance for such activities as studying, moving house, giving birth, growing old, looking after your health, or maintaining your car. If you worry about it, plan for it! But ensure that your planning does not become obsessive or a source of worry in itself; and don't over-plan for things that are unlikely to ever happen.

Develop confidence in your ability to cope with life

If you think that you lack the ability to cope with life's demands and stresses, then you are likely to worry about them happening. See page 58 for some thoughts on how to develop 'ability-confidence'. If there are things you frequently worry about, study them, learning as much as you can about them. Understanding the things you fear will give you more power over them and build confidence in your ability to cope.

Deal with any perfectionism

Do you tend to hold perfectionistic expectations about

solving life's problems? Watch for any absolutistic beliefs like: 'Every problem has a perfect solution and I must find it.' Perfection is impossible; but expecting it will keep you tense and anxious (and, paradoxically, will lower your productivity). Accept that there is never any one 'right' solution — just solutions that are better (or worse) than others.[2]

Work toward self-acceptance

Do you worry about criticism and disapproval from other people, or fear that if such-and-such occurs you will be shown to be deficient as a human being? *Self-image anxiety* (page 36) underlies much worrying. The solution is to develop self-acceptance. This involves uncovering any *demand* that you be something other than what you are (while still desiring to make any changes that may be in your interests). See page 80 for help with developing self-acceptance.

Finally, accept what you can't change

What if you can't change something you dislike? This is where acceptance of reality comes in. Acceptance is a way to cope with the realities of life when things don't — as they often won't — happen as we would wish. To accept something is to do three things:

1 *Acknowledge it exists:* see it as inevitable that many things will not be to your liking, and view uncertainty, frustration and disappointment as aspects of normal life.

2 *Believe there is no reason why it should not exist*: You may *prefer* people or things to be different from how they are (and you may even work at changing them) — but remind yourself that there is no law of the universe that says they *should* or *must* be different.

3 *See it as bearable:* acknowledge that you dislike some things, and find them unpleasant — but without catastrophising them into 'horrible' or 'unbearable'.

Some people have trouble with the idea of acceptance. They think that to accept something means they have to like it, agree with it, justify it, be indifferent to it, or resign themselves to it. But acceptance is none of these things. You can dislike something, see it as unjustified, and continue to prefer that it did not exist. You can be concerned about it. You can take action to change it, if change is possible. But you can still accept it by rejecting the notion that it *should* not exist and that it absolutely *must* be changed.

Acceptance can be summed up with a paraphrase of an old saying: 'Have the courage to change the things you can, the serenity to accept the things you can't — and the wisdom to know the difference.'

From worry to rational concern

Let's finish with the most important aspect of all: changing the self-defeating beliefs that maintain the worrying habit. Following is a collection of typical worry beliefs, along with a rational alternative to each.

Your formal self-help programme may end when your worrying has been reduced to a manageable level and you are facing all the things you were previously avoiding. Bear in mind, though, some return of worrying is almost certain, especially at times of stress. Expecting this to happen is the best protection from slipping back, because you will be prepared for it and ready to dust off your coping skills. If you are willing to help yourself in the future, worrying need never take control of your life again.

Denise got her worrying under control. Paul did too. He accepted that a lifetime of anticipating disaster would take

Worry beliefs	Concern beliefs
If I worry about things that might be dangerous, unpleasant or frightening, I can stop them happening.	Worrying about things that might go wrong won't stop them happening — but it will upset me now! Better to do what I can about the future, and then get on with living in the present.
There are certain things in life that I just can't stand.	Certain things are uncomfortable or unpleasant, but it's wrong to say I 'can't stand' them. If that were true, I wouldn't be here to tell the tale!
I should worry when other people have problems or feel unhappy.	I can't change other people's problems and bad feelings by getting myself upset.
It is 'caring' to worry — if I didn't worry, that would show I was an uncaring person.	Worrying has nothing to do with caring. Better I demonstrate caring in *action* rather than rumination!
If I feel anxious, this proves that something bad is likely to happen.	I feel because of what I *think*. Assuming that a feeling proves something about reality is just 'emotional reasoning'.
Life must be safe: my marriage, home, money, job, etc, must be totally guaranteed.	Safety is preferable — but in real life there are no guarantees. Making safety a 'must' (rather than a preference) will just keep me worrying about it.
Because I can't stand discomfort and pain, I must avoid them at all costs.	Total avoidance would mean a restricted life. Although I don't like discomfort and pain, I can bear them.
Every problem has an ideal solution, and I should not relax until I find it.	Problems usually have many possible solutions. The wisest thing is to select the best one available and get on with it (and accept reality when I can't have the ideal).

some work to overcome, and that he would probably never stop worrying completely. But reducing his apprehensiveness by 80 per cent made his (and his family's) life much happier. Whenever worrying returns, Denise and Paul dust off their worry diaries and stop the fear before it takes over. It has been more than worth the effort for them. It can be the same for you. So don't delay — start taking control of your worrying now!

Anger:
who controls who?

Of all the emotions that human beings have trouble controlling, anger seems to be the most likely to get out of hand. It also seems the most difficult to change. This is because it is based on a sense of one's 'rightness' — and who wants to give that up? Anger is not in itself a problematical emotion. In fact, anger has value when it serves as a motivator to seek change to circumstances we dislike. But it sometimes gets out of hand, taking over a person's reasoning faculties and leading to rage, hostility and destructive behaviour.

This was Ben's experience. His anger had been problematical since he was a child. Now, married to Nicola, with two young children and a small plumbing business he was struggling to get off the ground, his angry outbursts were putting his family and future at risk. This was the trigger that led him to at last realise he needed to start taking control.

What causes hostile anger?

Anger results from a combination of factors. Clearly the environment is involved, given that angry episodes usually have a situational trigger that sets them off. At a more fundamental level, one's biological make-up is also part of the picture. The most important factor, though, is psychological.

You may have noticed that you are more likely to feel angry when frustrated in some way. Frustration is a normal reaction when a person fails to get something they want, or gets something they don't want. Probably all human beings are subject to frustration every day of their lives, and people mostly take it in their stride.

In Ben's case, however, his frustration was leading to *hostile* anger: rage directed at people rather than at the problems. Hostile anger occurs when a person fails to get what they think they *need* or *must* or *should* have. Such anger is an emotional response to a frustrated *demand* (as opposed to a frustrated *preference*).

If you ask someone with an anger problem what causes their ill temper, they will usually have a simple answer: 'other people'. But this raises two questions. How can an *external* event create an *internal* reaction? And why is it that one person can be disappointed but calm in the face of a circumstance to which another, such as Ben, reacts with rage? In reality, events and circumstances alone do not cause anger. Anger results from how people *view* what happens to them. Dysfunctional anger typically arises from distorted *perceptions* and the self-defeating *evaluations* that follow.

Some of the material that follows has appeared in earlier chapters, but here we will study it within the specific context of anger.

Distorted perceptions

We are constantly perceiving what is going on around us and drawing interpretations, or 'inferences'. As we saw earlier in the book (see page 42), there are certain ways of perceiving that result in distorted, inaccurate views of reality. Here are the most common ones:

- *Mind-reading:* believing that you know what is going on in another person's mind — for example, inferring that someone thinks badly of you. Ben, for instance, sometimes interpreted his wife's behaviour as showing that she did not respect him (which she denied).

- *Fortune-telling:* believing your own predictions of the future — for example, 'If I don't get my partner under control then he/she might leave me.'

- *Over-generalisation:* building up something in your mind so that it becomes bigger than it really is — for example, 'Everything is going wrong in my life.'

- *Filtering:* seeing only the negatives — 'there's nothing good about my life/this situation/this person/etc.'

- *Emotional reasoning:* believing that because you *feel* angry this *proves* that someone has done wrong — for example, 'I *know* that he/she has done something wrong — otherwise I wouldn't be angry!' This is a common way of thinking for people with anger problems. Ben engaged in emotional reasoning whenever he thought that, because he *felt* angry with his children, customers or suppliers, this was *proof* that they had behaved badly.

Self-defeating evaluations

Misinterpretations alone, though, are not enough to cause emotional responses. The real cause is the *evaluations* that we apply to our inferences. There are four ways human beings typically evaluate their experiences that create emotional disturbance and dysfunctional behaviour:

- *Demanding.* We all have expectations about how we want the world and the people in it to be. Hostile anger results when our preferences are escalated into *demands*. Demanding comes in two flavours: (a) *moralising* about how people 'should' or 'should not' behave; and (b) *musturbation:* believing that the world or one's circumstances 'have' to or 'need' to be a certain way.

- *Can't-stand-it-itis* refers to where demands directed outwards typically lead to *low frustration tolerance* or *discomfort intolerance*, where events and circumstances are viewed as 'unbearable', 'intolerable' or 'un-stand-able'.

- *Awfulising* refers to evaluating an event or circumstance as the 'worst that could happen'. Anger frequently results from anxiety, and violence often represents an attempt to ward off perceived threats. Such threats may be of two types: (1) perceived threats to well-being (discomfort anxiety); and perceived threats to self-image (self-image or 'ego' anxiety).

- *People rating* refers to the practice of globally evaluating people — for example, labelling a person as a 'bitch', 'bastard', or in some other all-encompassing way that makes it easier to be angry with them.

Demanding may be the key type of evaluative thinking, with the other three deriving from it. For example, we only think something is 'awful' or 'unbearable' because we demand that it not happen; or we evaluate ourselves as 'failures' only because we demand that we always succeed and never fail at anything important.

Ben, unfortunately, had grown up with a tendency to view the world around him — and himself — in terms of rigid demands. He was highly moralistic, with fixed ideas about how people should behave. Although he often felt guilty for letting his anger get out of control (as he put it, 'I let myself down'), he nevertheless believed that his problems were mainly the result of other people not behaving as they 'should'. When he then evaluated their actions as 'intolerable', he further fuelled his rage by defining the others as 'bad' or 'stupid'.

Core beliefs

Underlying our surface thinking or 'automatic thoughts' is a set of assumptions and rules about the world: 'core beliefs' that have their origin in childhood learning and are almost always held subconsciously. The inferences we draw and how we evaluate them are determined by our particular underlying beliefs. Here are some typical core beliefs that tend to be associated with anger:

1 Others must never do anything to devalue me.

2 I should be able to have the things I want, and live my life as I choose.

3 Other people must never behave in ways that frustrate or deprive me, or upset the stability of my life.

4 The only way to get people to change their behaviour is to get angry with them.

5 People should always behave in a correct and right fashion.

6 People who behave badly are bad people — and they deserve blame and punishment.

7 To be a real, genuine human being, you must always let your feelings show.

8 Anger is evil and destructive.

Ben held core beliefs similar to 1, 3, 4 and 5. Belief 3

provides a vivid illustration of the way in which underlying core beliefs determine what one thinks in specific situations. Holding this belief made Ben hypersensitive to anything that might be a threat to his comfort or stability, and thus made him more likely to *misinterpret* the behaviour of others and then to *evaluate* the threat as 'awful' or 'unbearable'.

The ABC model

The way in which thinking creates anger can be illustrated using the ABC model we saw in Chapter 1.[1] Below is given an example, drawn from Ben's experience.

A. Activating event (experience, event or situation that started things off):
Children playing noisily, could not hear television programme.

B. Beliefs (self-talk that led from **A** to **C**):
Underlying core belief:
Others should never do things that frustrate me or upset my life, and when they do, I must get them under control.
Thoughts specific to the situation (but arising out of the core belief):
Perception: They are out of control.
Evaluations: This is intolerable — I can't stand it.
I have to make them behave.

C. Consequence (reaction to the **A**):
Physiological signs: Got very tense.
Emotions: Felt angry.
Behaviours: Went into lounge, shouted at children and called them abusive names.

Other causes

Although anger results primarily from thinking processes, *physiological causes* (such as tension, agitation or ill-humour) can aggravate the emotion. Also, if a person lacks coping skills in areas such as assertiveness, communication or problem-solving, they may tend to fall back on anger to manage what life throws at them. An effective approach to anger management will take all factors into account.

How to take charge of your anger

As we have seen, anger results from a combination of factors: biological, situational and psychological. Change in any of these areas can be used to reduce problematical anger. Most benefit will follow from focussing on change on the psychological area — in particular, on change in the thinking that creates specific episodes of anger.

Do you want to combat unhelpful anger directed at people and replace it with moderate, functional anger directed at solving problems? This would involve raising your tolerance for frustration, through a programme such as the following:

1 First, assess the problem and identify the causes that are applicable to you.

2 Introduce yourself to some new ways of viewing anger.

3 Develop some important coping techniques to help you manage both internal emotions and external life problems: re-thinking, controlling physical symptoms, and effective communication with other people.

4 Practise these skills via planned, graduated exposure to anger triggers that challenges your coping abilities but does not overwhelm them.

Assess your anger and its causes

Change is more likely to happen effectively and efficiently if you first identify your motivation for change, your personal anger patterns, and any functions that anger serves for you that could hinder you from changing.

Check out your motivation for change

Do you see your anger as inappropriate? If you think that your angry reactions are not the problem and that other people or circumstances need to change, then the rest of this chapter will probably not be relevant to you. Personal change will be your agenda, however, if you have come to the following conclusions:

1 My current experience of anger is not in my interests.

2 The cause of my anger is within myself, not outside.

3 If I do the work, change is within my power.

Even though you may already be willing to change, it will still be useful to articulate why such change is in your interests. List your reasons: this information will give you something to fall back on when the process of change becomes uncomfortable and you are tempted to give up.

Consider where your anger started

It is sometimes useful to understand where your learning regarding anger may have come from. Ask yourself questions like the following:

- How did my father/mother/siblings behave, and how did I know they were angry? Was there any violence or verbal/passive aggression?

- What messages did I get from my parents about the

expression of anger — OK or not OK? How did I know it was OK or not OK?

Don't, however, fall into the trap of spending too much time on the past. Your focus needs to be on the *current* causes of your anger.

Identify the current causes

Become aware of the *activating events* that trigger your angry episodes, and the *consequences* (how you feel and behave). The purpose is for you to learn to recognise these signs at an early stage when anger is coming on, so that you can take action before your brain shuts down. A useful way to identify these signs is to keep a diary of **A**s and **C**s for a few weeks.

Here is an example, from Ben's experience, of such a diary:

A. Activating event	C. Consequence
Children noisy, couldn't hear TV programme.	Got tense. Felt angry. Shouted at them and abused them.
Partner arguing about money.	Mad 7/10. Stormed off in car.

As (*activating events*) — the persons, situations and states that trigger anger — might include such things as perceived rejection or rule-breaking by others, arguments, alcohol use, or feeling anxious (you may react to your own internal emotional states as well as to external events). You can also use the information from your diary to check out what might be the gains you get from becoming angry (for example, it seems to release tension or frustration, or helps you 'control' other people, and the like).

To identify your **C**s (*consequences*) — the physical

sensations, emotional states and behaviours that occur when you are angry — look for:

- *body signals* — becoming tense and aroused, feeling anxious, stomach aching, sweating or feeling unusually cold, breathing speeding up, head aching, back aching, and so on

- *behaviours* — becoming mean, blaming others, using sarcasm or forced humour, feeling depressed, withdrawing, acting over-nice and trying to please, going quiet, becoming verbally or physically violent, changes in eating or sleeping patterns, etc.

When you have become used to recording the **A**s and **C**s, extend the diary to include the **B**s — the thoughts that are activated by the **A**s. Remember: **A** does not cause **C**. Events and circumstances that occur activate your *thinking* — this then creates your emotional and behavioural reaction.

A. Activating event	B. Beliefs/thoughts	C. Consequence
Children noisy, couldn't hear TV programme.	They are out of control. I can't stand it. I have to make them behave.	Got tense. Felt angry. Shouted at them and abused them.
Partner arguing about money.	She shouldn't tell me what to do. She's a demanding bitch.	Mad 7/10. Stormed off in car.

How do you view anger?

Before you proceed with your self-help programme, it might be important to examine a few ways of viewing anger so that you clarify what to aim for, and keep your own problem in perspective.

First, it is important to see that there is a difference between what you *feel* (the emotion of anger) and what you *do* (the aggressive verbal and physical actions directed at people or property). You can *feel* angry without needing to *act* on it.

Secondly, anger in itself is not 'evil'; it can be destructive or constructive. Accordingly, identify and deal with any secondary disturbance about having an anger problem — especially guilt, which simply perpetuates anger. If you engage in guilty self-downing — telling yourself 'Because I have this anger problem, I am a rotten, useless bitch/ bastard' — what message are you giving yourself about your ability to change? View anger in practical terms — that is, in terms of its consequences — rather than as a 'moral' issue; and accept your*self* while rejecting your angry *behaviour*. See page 80 for more guidance on self-acceptance and how to achieve it.

Finally, it is helpful to see anger as having three different forms — passive, aggressive and constructive:

1 *Passive* anger is hostility that is expressed indirectly or covertly, often by omission. Going silent, withdrawing, impatience, being late, 'forgetting' to do things, or denying sex or physical affection are all ways that a person may express passive anger. Unfortunately, it blocks them from seeking constructive change in the situations to which they are reacting.

2 *Aggressive* hostility is more overt and involves verbal or physical violence (against people or things). It sometimes leads to dangerous risk-taking (such as, for example, when a person is enraged while driving).

3 *Constructive* anger is very different. It involves moderate emotions, such as irritation, annoyance, dissatisfaction, displeasure and disappointment. These are

still angry feelings, but they will not cause people to lose their heads. Most importantly, constructive anger is directed against unwanted events and circumstances — not against people. It leads to problem-solving rather than people-harming.

Re-think your anger

Now it is time to turn to the strategies that will help you achieve change. We will start with the most important skill you will need to keep anger under control: how to identify and change the self-defeating beliefs that create and maintain it.

Rational self-analysis

After a week or so of recording the ABC diary described earlier, extend it to include: **D** — disputing self-defeating beliefs; **E** — developing a new emotional and behavioural goal; and **F** — further action you will take to reinforce the new ways of thinking developed with the analysis.[2] Note that it is usually most effective to proceed with an analysis in the following order: **A**, **C**, **B**, **E**, **D**, **F**. Here is Ben's analysis as an example.

A. **Activating event** (what started things off):
Children playing noisily, could not hear television programme.

B. **Beliefs** (what I told myself about the **A**):
Thoughts specific to the situation:

1. They are out of control.

2. I can't stand it.

3. I have to make them behave.

Underlying core belief:
Others should never do things that frustrate or upset me; when they do, I must get them under control.

C. Consequence (how I felt and/or behaved):

Emotions: Felt angry.

Behaviours: Went into lounge, shouted at children and called them abusive names.

E. New Effect (how I would prefer to feel/behave):
I would prefer to feel annoyed rather than hostile; and calmly explain that I like to relax after work, and ask them to play more quietly.

D. Disputation and new beliefs (that will help me achieve the new Effect I want):

1. They are not out of control — they are just playing.

2. Even if they were out of control, I wouldn't like it, but I could survive it.

3. It would be helpful to train them to behave, but telling myself I 'have' to only makes me lose control — and that doesn't model the good behaviour I want to teach my children.

4. I would prefer others not to do things I dislike, but where is it written that they 'must' not? And, anyway, others don't frustrate me — I frustrate myself with what I think about their behaviour. And thinking that I 'have' to control them only leads me to get out of control!

F. Further action (what I will do to avoid the same dysfunctional thinking and reactions in future):

1. Re-read the material on demanding.

2. Apologise to the kids now.

3. Over the next week, record my favourite TV programmes and pick times to watch them when the kids are playing in the lounge (in order to practise tolerating their noise).

The daily thought record

The daily thought record is an alternative to rational self-analysis that achieves a similar purpose in a more succinct format, and it may be useful in the early stages of your self-help programme when you need to identify and change irrational thinking on a frequent basis. It is an extension of the ABC diary shown earlier (see next page).

Whichever approach is used, self-analysis with anger problems will usually involve:

- challenging demands directed at other people or the world

- developing acceptance of people (but not necessarily their behaviour)

- putting unwanted events and circumstances into perspective rather than catastrophising them.

How to dispute

At the end of this chapter is a list of beliefs typically involved with angry reactions, along with rational alternatives. Before you substitute a new belief, however, it is important to effectively dispute and deal with the old one. Effective disputation, as described earlier in the book (see page 74), involves the use of three key questions:

1 *Is this belief helpful or harmful?* Ask yourself: 'How does this belief affect me? Does it help me keep my

Daily thought record

A. Activating event	B. Beliefs/thoughts	C. Consequence	D. Disputation/rational response	E. New effect	F. Further action
Children noisy, couldn't hear TV.	They're out of control. I can't stand it.	Got tense. Felt angry. Shouted at kids & abused them.	They're not out of control — they're just playing. I don't like it, but I can stand it.	Felt annoyed but calmer.	Re-read material on demanding. Apologise to kids.
Partner arguing about money.	She shouldn't tell me what to do. She's a demanding bitch.	Mad 7/10. Stormed off in car.	Why shouldn't she have an opinion on how the money is spent? She's not demanding — she's just worried about how we are going to make ends meet.	Felt concerned.	Read rational card. Set a time to talk about the issue.

head and engage in constructive problem-solving, or does it make me fall out of my tree?' When you can clearly see that a particular belief leads to negative emotional and behavioural consequences for you, you will be more motivated to change it.

2 *What does the evidence say?* Ask yourself questions like: 'What is the evidence for and against this belief?' 'Where is it written that ... ?' and the like.

3 *Does it follow?* Check whether the belief logically follows from the facts. Ask questions like: 'How does it follow that because I would *like* the children to keep quiet, therefore they absolutely *must*?' or 'How does this thing that is *uncomfortable* become something I *can't stand*?'

Motivating yourself: the 'benefits calculation'

Given that anger is such a difficult emotion to change, how can you increase your motivation to change? A useful way to do this is with the 'benefits calculation'. To complete such a calculation, follow these steps:

1 Either draw four boxes on one large sheet of paper, or use four separate sheets.

2 List all the advantages and disadvantages of continuing to behave in the old angry way.

3 Do the same with the new replacement behaviour you wish to consolidate.

4 Decide how much value or benefit each item has for you, negatively or positively, then add up the pros and cons.

The example on the next page is based on Ben's issue of anger in the family situation.

Keep getting enraged ◄— MY OPTIONS —► Learn to control my anger.

Advantages	I feel superior.	4	People will like me more.	7
	They usually go quiet.	5	Less shouting in the house.	7
	They are more careful around me.	4	I won't lose the family.	10
		+13		+24
Disadvantages	People dislike me.	7	Will be hard to control the urge to shout.	5
	Afterwards, I don't like myself.	8		
	They are only careful for a while, then they go back to the old ways.	6	It will take more time to fix problems.	4
			I will miss the high I get.	3
		−21		−12
	Overall total:	**−8**	Overall total:	**+12**

Note that the advantages to the first option will often represent disadvantages to the second option, and *vice versa*.

This may seem like doubling up, but it actually aids clarification.

How to combat awfulising

A useful way to get awfulising into perspective is to complete a 'catastrophe scale'. For instructions, see page 81. An example from Ben's experience is given at the top of the next page.

Keep the chart and add to it from time to time. Whenever you are upset about something, ascertain what 'badness-rating' you are giving it and pencil it on your chart, then see how it compares to the items already there. Soon, you will realise you have been exaggerating the badness involved and move the item down the list until it is in perspective.

	Ben's catastrophe scale	
	Event: Nicola messed up the cheque book again.	
100	Burning alive	original placing
90	Losing my family	2nd placing
80	Becoming a paraplegic	3rd placing
70	Being diagnosed with cancer	
60	Losing my business	
50	House getting burgled	
40	Having my car stolen	
30	Losing my wallet	
20	***Nicola messing up the cheque book***	final placing
10	Catching a cold	
5	Missing my favourite TV programme	
0	Having a coffee at home	

Manage the physical causes

While changing the beliefs that cause anger is the priority, it will also help to reduce any tension and ill-humour that may exacerbate the anger. Depending on what your assessment showed, strategies that you might pursue include:

- reducing tension via relaxation training (page 169)

- anxiety management[3]

- moderation of alcohol use, and no alcohol at all when angry or upset (you will also benefit from reducing your caffeine intake if you drink more than five cups a day) — see Chapter 9 for more information.

Physiological strategies are 'palliative' — that is, they ease the symptoms without addressing the causes — but are a useful adjunct to your self-help armoury.

Develop additional skills as needed

Some people will need additional skills training in how to use anger adaptively rather than destructively. The idea is to learn how to minimise the dysfunctional aspects of anger, and instead engage in problem-solving behaviour.

Time out

Are your angry responses leading to aggressive behaviour that puts you or others at risk? If so, 'time out' may be a wise strategy, especially in the early stages of therapy before you have learned to deal with the underlying cause of your anger. The instructions are as follows.

Begin by preparing the scene: explain to your partner what you will do when you feel anger in future, and arrange to have their cooperation. Whenever you identify the early stages of anger, follow these steps:

1 Share with your partner that you are feeling angry, and say you are going to take time out.

2 Leave the situation for about one hour. Avoid drinking or driving while angry; instead, do something physical (brisk walk, run, gardening, etc) and/or do a *self-analysis* to deal with the self-defeating thinking involved.

3 When the hour is up, return and check in with your partner and offer to talk about what happened.

Communication and assertiveness training

It is possible to change things you dislike without using anger. This involves communicating with others effectively so that you are able to ask for what you want and say 'no' to what you don't. If you think that developing these skills would be helpful for you, see Chapter 13 for guidance.

Problem-solving training

If you know how to use task-oriented, problem-solving strategies, you will be able to deal with problems straight away rather than bottling up your feelings. A problem-solving model is described in detail in Chapter 19.

Practise your coping skills with controlled exposure

The final step is to apply what you have learned. Rather than simply promising yourself that from now on you will handle things differently, it will most likely be more effective (and safer) to practise your new skills in a graduated fashion and under controlled circumstances. What follows is a process for doing this.[4]

Step 1. Develop a hierarchy

Start by listing anger situations you are likely to meet in real life (you may have already done this if you kept the ABC diary described earlier in this chapter). Rate the level of anger you would associate with each situation, then order the list into a hierarchy according to the anger rating for each item. An example of a hierarchy developed by Ben is given at the top of the next page.

Step 2. Exposure via imagery

Before confronting the listed situations in real life, confront them in your imagination, where you can safely practise your coping skills. Progressively using each hierarchy scene (starting from the lowest scene in the hierarchy and moving up), expose yourself to manageable doses of the anger triggers by vividly imagining yourself

Anger level:	Exposure task:
10	Talk with Nicola about our finances.
9	Record my favourite programme, then watch it while the kids are playing.
8	Go shopping with Nicola.
7	Ask Nicola's opinion on the new political party.
6	Watch TV news.
5	Go into the lounge when I know all the kids' toys will be everywhere on the floor.
4	Talk to the guy at work who supports that new political party.

in the situation involved. Use techniques such as rational-emotive imagery (page 83) or rational self-analysis (page 70) to identify and dispute the thoughts that create the anger you feel while carrying out the exercise. In addition, use any other coping techniques relevant to you — for example, deep-muscle relaxation — in order to reduce any tension or other physical symptoms that may exacerbate the anger.

Step 3. Exposure in real-life situations

When you are ready, move on to real-life exposure. Progressively confront the situations on your list, as you did in step 2, except this time in real life. While engaging in the exposure, inhibit your usual response (for example, argumentativeness, defensiveness, demanding of others, etc) and instead use the new strategies you have developed.

The purpose of exposure is to give you practice at increasing your frustration tolerance and coping in a non-hostile way with a variety of situations, where the practice is under your control (see page 87 for more information on the technique of controlled exposure).

Finishing your programme

Your formal self-help programme comes to an end when you are satisfied that the targets you set have been achieved to a level where you will be able to maintain them in the long term. Ensure that you are prepared to cope with setbacks and know what to do when angry reactions return, as they most likely will. From here on, as with most of the other control areas discussed in this book, it is a matter of 'management, not cure'. If you are prepared to dust off your coping skills from time to time throughout your life, then you can look forward to a lifetime where you control your anger, rather than letting the anger control you.

A sample of anger-creating irrational beliefs

Hostile anger beliefs	Constructive anger alternatives
Others must never do anything to devalue me.	The actions of others can't 'devalue' me. I don't magically change because of what others say or do.
I should be able to have the things I want, and live my life as I choose.	It's OK to want things my way (and to try to achieve it), but there is no law of the universe that says I *should* or *must* get what I want how I want it.
I can't stand it when people get in my way.	It's disappointing when people get in my way, but I can stand it — especially if I avoid demanding and catastrophising.
Other people should never behave in ways that frustrate or deprive me, or upset the stability of my existence.	I'd prefer it if people didn't do things I dislike. But, in real life, they sometimes do! Anyway, it's not their actions that frustrate me — it's my own demanding thoughts.
If the world were a better place, I wouldn't need to get upset.	Unfortunately, the world is not a better place. But I can avoid getting upset about this fact by changing the way I view it.
If I didn't get mad, things would never change.	Getting mad disables me. I'm more likely to change things by keeping my head and being assertive rather than aggressive.

(Continued)

Hostile anger beliefs	Constructive anger alternatives
People should always behave in a correct and right fashion.	In real life, people don't always behave correctly. No amount of demanding is going to make this reality go away. Anyway, who decides what's right?
People who behave badly are bad people — and they deserve blame and punishment.	People are not what they do. Behaving badly doesn't make someone a bad person — it just shows they are a person who sometimes behaves badly.
People only do things to frustrate me.	Am I a god, that I can see into the inner recesses of others' minds and discern their motivations?
I wouldn t be human if I didn't lose my cool.	Just because something is human doesn't make it desirable. Anyway, to be reasonable and understand someone else's viewpoint is also human.
Anger is evil and destructive.	Anger is neither good nor bad — it's just an emotion. I can choose to express it constructively rather than destructively.

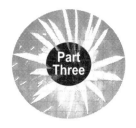

Part Three

Control
over your body

Human beings are complex: we are not just mind, nor just body — the two are intimately linked. (As we shall see later, we are also part of the wider environment in which we live.) This book takes a bio-psycho-social approach, working on the assumption that exercising control over all three areas of our being and existence is more likely to lead to a happy life.

Part Three will show you how to take control over the physical side of your existence, in particular: your health (what you take into your body and how you exercise it); knowing how to let go of the tension that may be tightening you up at the wrong times; and overcoming that all-too-common affliction of modern life, sleeplessness.

Each chapter in this and the next part of the book will follow a similar format: first, a description of the problem, then the presentation of solutions, and finally a discussion of the most common reasons why people may not apply the solutions, along with suggestions for overcoming these blocks.

9

Healthy living:
make your own prescription

Feeling good involves body as well as mind. Abusing the body creates distress, not necessarily in the short term but often later and longer; conversely, we can make ourselves feel good by eating well, exercising and avoiding dangerous behaviour.

When your body is reacting to stress, biochemical changes occur which have implications for your patterns of eating and exercising. For example, when stressed, your immune system is less able to protect you against the bugs and chemicals to which you are exposed in day-to-day life. You can help yourself at such times of extra stress by paying extra attention to exercise and what you eat and drink. Unfortunately, many people under stress do the opposite — they stop their usual exercise or allow their dietary standards to fall. For instance, a grieving person might eat less, or someone under extra pressure at work might increase their intake of caffeine.

This was the road down which Michael was heading. His employer had promoted him from software engineer to leader of his team. In his mid-thirties with a growing family to support and a mortgage to repay, the extra money had been welcome. A year later, however, he was not so happy. Michael had discovered that being a good engineer did not mean he possessed all the skills needed for management.

Stress was becoming a constant companion. Unfortunately, in trying to cope, he had developed some bad habits that were making matters worse. Thinking that spending more time at work would help, Michael had stopped going to the gym and spent less time outdoors with his family. He had lost count of how much coffee he was drinking, and found that he was hoarding small change in order to feed the machine at work that dispensed candy bars.

The problem

There are many ways in which bad nutritional practice can create distress:

- *Caffeine* stimulates production of adrenalin, which raises heart rate and blood pressure and irritates the linings of the stomach and intestines. Excess caffeine keeps the body's chemistry 'on edge', making a person more likely to react to things that happen around them, as well as causing headaches and sleep problems. As few as five caffeine drinks a day can produce these symptoms.

- *Nicotine* has a mixed effect. In the short term it may relax, but later it raises the heart rate. Its addictive nature will also create agitation when a cigarette is not available. Nicotine is one of the most addictive substances known to humankind, because of the speed at which it affects the brain.

- *Sugar* can increase energy levels in the short term, but the boost is temporary because the body reacts by secreting insulin to hold down the amount of sugar in the bloodstream. The insulin tends to keep acting after it has normalised the blood-sugar level, causing a drop in energy. A diet which includes an excessive intake of pure sugar raises insulin levels to the extent of causing fatigue, headaches, restlessness and difficulty thinking clearly.

- *Alcohol abuse*, as well as the numerous social problems it creates, often leads to poor nutrition, liver damage and excess weight. It can create low blood sugar, increase blood pressure, damage the heart, and injure the stomach and gastrointestinal linings. Being a diuretic, it can compound the body's tendency to dehydrate when stressed.

- *Extreme dieting* places a lot of stress on the body. If you radically reduce your food intake, the body will automatically gear up to counter the threat to its equilibrium. It will slow down its functioning and burn calories at a lower rate to compensate for the shortage of fuel. The percentage of body fat will also increase, which means the body needs fewer calories than before the diet began. If you return to a normal food intake, you will gain weight on fewer calories than before.

Michael's nutritional problems were too much sugar and caffeine, which gave him a temporary boost but left him feeling tired when the fix wore off, coupled with rushed or missed meals, often too close to bed-time (if at all). For much of each workday he felt tense, and was concerned that this was increasingly the case at home. His sleep was beginning to suffer.

The good news

A diet that contains all the nutrients your body needs will defend you more effectively against distress. At times of extra stress, such as work overload, bereavement, surgery or an accident, a balanced diet will provide protection and aid recovery.

Exercise also helps in many ways. It elevates mood by increasing blood flow and releasing hormones that stimulate the brain and nervous system. Exercise increases muscle functioning, improves oxygen delivery to the body, reduces blood pressure, and can improve the functioning of the immune system and help relieve headaches and asthma. It aids relaxation by decreasing tension in the muscles, and improves sleep. People who engage in moderate exercise on a regular basis are less prone to abuse substances or use other unhealthy ways to cope with stress.

Eat to feel good

Good nutrition practices will help you avoid unnecessary stress on your body. Shortly we will see how you can give your body some extra help at times of increased stress; but first let's start with the basics of everyday nutrition.

- *Have regular, set meal times.* Avoid snatching meals — allow enough time to eat without rushing. Make your meal times a priority. Don't eat a big meal late in the evening, or your digestion will be working overtime when you are trying to sleep. Have breakfast every day — a lot of people skip what dieticians say is the most important meal of all. And, if it works for you, it is fine to eat a number of small meals through the day rather than the standard three big ones.

- *Don't eat more than you need.* If you find yourself putting on weight, you may be eating more than your body requires. Eat less or exercise more.

- *Maintain a low fat intake.* Keep your total fat intake low, and as far as possible take it in polyunsaturated form (vegetable oils and some fish oils) rather than saturated (red meat, hard cheese, cream, eggs, butter, fried foods and many convenience foods).

- *Use sugar and salt sparingly.* Try to buy products without added sugar and salt. Minimise your consumption of convenience and takeaway foods which often have high levels of sugar, fat and salt, as do luncheon meats and bacon.

- *Use alcohol in moderation.* A standard drink is 200 ml of beer, a small glass of wine, or one measure of spirits. Women need to keep their intake within 14 drinks in any one week, or three in any one session. For men, these totals are 21 and six, respectively. Note that these levels are *maximums*, so you would be well advised to keep your normal intake considerably lower. The US Department of Health and Human Services, for instance, defines moderate drinking as no more that one drink per day for women and three for men.[1] If you are driving, New Zealand Ministry of Health guidelines suggest no more than two drinks for women and three for men[2] (for some people these levels may need to be even lower; note, also, that these guidelines could change, depending on changes in legislation). Drink slowly — one drink an hour is the limit your liver can handle. Always eat when you drink; food delays the absorption of alcohol into your bloodstream.

- *Get as much fibre as possible.* Sources include wholegrain bread, fibre-rich breakfast cereals and the skins of fruits and vegetables. Fibre helps to lower raised cholesterol in the body.

- *Drink lots of water.* Water is the best fluid to drink

throughout the day. It contains none of the sugars present in soft drinks and to some extent in fruit juice. You need about six to eight glasses of fluid each day — more when you exercise. Water helps fibre do its good work by bulking it out, provides the cells with fluid, and helps the kidneys flush out waste products.

- *Eat a lot of fruit and vegetables,* especially dark green, leafy vegetables. Get them fresh as much as possible, eat them raw when you can, steam them rather than boil, or boil them only lightly. Fruit and vegetables contain many antioxidants, which help the immune system.

- *Favour whole, unprocessed foods* — wholegrain breads and cereals, dried beans and peas, fresh fruits and vegetables, lean meats, poultry, seafood, non-fat or low-fat milk and cheeses.

Special nutrition for times of extra stress

When the body is more stressed than usual, it uses greater amounts of energy, drawn from the principal sources of protein, fat, carbohydrates and vitamins. You need to maintain your food intake and not fall into the common trap of eating less because your appetite is diminished.

- Keep up your intake of:
  - —*Carbohydrate foods* — bread, pasta, potatoes, etc.
  - —*Vitamins* — C (citrus fruits, berries, broccoli, tomatoes), A (silverbeet, broccoli, carrots, pumpkin, apricots) and E (nuts, seeds, vegetable oils, wholegrain breads and cereals).
  - —*Minerals* — calcium (silverbeet, broccoli, pumpkin), zinc and iron (red meat, dark poultry meat, dark

green, leafy vegetables, dry beans and peas, whole grains, potatoes, dried fruit, berries and nuts).

- Avoid foods high in salt — they will elevate your blood pressure.

- Keep your meals as regular as possible. Try to make meal times relaxing. If you have trouble eating large meals, it may help to eat more frequently, with small meals and snacks throughout the day.

- Finally, don't attempt to operate on a weight-reduction diet plan at times of extra stress, except with proper medical advice.

Getting dietary advice

The suggestions for good nutrition put forward in this chapter are necessarily very brief. You can get good advice (and bad advice too, unfortunately!) from numerous books and the Internet. Look for books that are written by professionally-qualified dieticians, or Internet sites connected with reputable health organisations. You may also, if you have special needs, benefit from consulting a professional dietician — your doctor could refer you if necessary.

One final caution: if you are taking prescribed medications, or have any health problem that might preclude you from eating certain foods, check with your doctor before making any significant changes to your diet.

Exercise your body

Exercise, like healthy eating, can help you both avoid distress and cope better at times of extra stress. Before starting, it may be advisable to seek medical advice, especially if you are over 35, have heart trouble, pains in the chest, dizzy spells, high blood pressure, or bone or joint problems.

To keep motivated, do exercises you find enjoyable and which suit your personality type. What do you prefer — competitive or non-competitive activities, exercising with others or alone, exercise that requires a lot of concentration or only a little?

Develop a programme that is realistic given your circumstances, age and current level of fitness. There is one form of exercise that most people will be able to engage in — walking. It is good for the mind and body, requires no specialised equipment, you don't have to dress up for it, you can wear a headset to enjoy music at the same time, and it gets you out of the house or office. Increase the cardiovascular benefits by gradually walking faster and swinging your arms.

Two types of exercise are needed. *Aerobic* exercise keeps the cardiovascular system fit. It needs to be intense enough to raise your heart rate for 20 minutes at least three times per week. You can get this from jogging, cycling, swimming or walking fast. *Flexing* exercises keep the body supple. The aim is to put each joint through its full range of movement at least once during the session. Stretching exercises are the most common. Design a programme that includes both aerobic and flexing exercise.

Start your programme gradually. Straining your body could be dangerous, so don't push yourself or force your body to the point where it hurts. You will find that you can go further as your body becomes fitter and more supple. If you experience chest or muscular pain or any other distress, stop what you are doing and consult your doctor.

Exercise often — every second day at least. It is far better to exercise for 20 minutes each day than for 140 minutes once a week.

Keep up your exercise routine at times of extra stress

When things are rough, you may be tempted to skip exercise — at a time when you need it more than ever. If you feel stressed, put your headphones on and get walking. No time? Exercising will increase your efficiency, so the time spent will most likely be saved with interest.

Avoid dangerous behaviour

Unfortunately, it is possible to take a good thing too far. As you work to improve your nutrition and fitness, ensure that you avoid such extremes as the following.

- *Radical dieting.* Extreme diets can severely stress the body. Such dieting is usually undertaken for the wrong reasons, most often as part of a health fad or because of an obsession with one's body image. Don't go on a special diet without consulting a qualified health professional. Check if you really do need the diet. If you do, explore different ways to go about it and choose the safest.

- *Over-exercising.* It is possible for a person to become addicted to their adrenalin, or compulsively use exercise to avoid facing up to unhappiness in their life. Unfortunately, overexertion can create its own distress. Fatigue can lead to sleep problems, anxiety and depression, and the time spent on obsessive exercise will disrupt other areas of life.

If you find that exercise is becoming compulsive and taking over, cut back. You will feel uncomfortable at first, but this will pass. Replace the time with other, rewarding activities. If you can't break the addiction alone, seek help (see Chapter 21).

A programme to change your self-care habits

Now it's time to put the theory into practice. You will find it easier to achieve the goal of healthy living if you develop a series of steps to take you there, like the suggested outline that follows.

- **Step 1. Start by identifying your problems**

  Keep an 'eating and activity' log for about a week. Record the day, time, problematical activity (food/drink/smoking/exercising) and how much, where and with whom, what you were feeling and what you were thinking at the time. You could lay out your log something like this:

Date/time	Situation I was in	What I ate/drank/did	How I was feeling at the time
Sun 2.00pm	At home alone	2 cream doughnuts	Bored
Tue 6.30pm	At home, neighbours in their front garden	Watched TV instead of going for a walk as planned	Anxious about being seen in my shorts

- **Step 2. Evaluate what the log shows**

  Think about and list the things that are problematical for you.

- **Step 3. Design corrective actions**

  Some examples of problems and possible solutions are shown in the next section. Specify your aims as measurable behaviours. For example, 'Eat breakfast every morning', 'Keep within three standard drinks of alcohol per day', 'Stop smoking by …', 'Eat fruit instead of sweets' or 'Walk for 20 minutes every second day.'

- **Step 4. Be clear about your reasons**
  Write down the advantages of changing. When the going gets tough, you can remind yourself why you are doing it.

- **Step 5. Identify and deal with any blocks**
  Does your eating and activity log show any potential blocks? Design solutions, using the ideas explored in the previous two sections and the remainder of this chapter.

Michael, the stressed software engineer turned team leader, identified his health problems as too much caffeine (more than 20 cups of coffee most days), too many candy bars, missed meals and lack of exercise. He developed the following plan:

1 Reduce coffee to 16 cups per day for a week, then 12, then 8, until I am drinking no more than 5 cups per day. Increasingly replace coffee with water.

2 No more than one candy bar per half-day for a week, then one per day maximum. Take fresh fruit to work each day and eat it when I feel any craving for sweets.

3 Go home in time to eat dinner with the family at least four out of five working days.

4 Go to the gym once-weekly for a month, then increase to twice-weekly.

5 Work only one weekend day per month maximum, and every weekend have an outing with the family that involves physical activity.

(Michael had other issues needing attention, such as workload management, balancing work and home life, and dealing with other people. The solutions to these will be the subject of later chapters.)

Some examples of problems and solutions

Problems	Solutions
Excessive high-energy foods.	Reduce to guideline levels.
Biscuits, sweets, desserts.	Eat foods like fruit or yoghurt instead.
Fat or oil.	Use other cooking methods, such as baking or microwaving.
Snacks during the day.	Avoid too much snacking — try drinking water, or doing something physical.
Eating to improve mood.	Do something else to improve your mood when you feel bored or low: exercise, walk, talk to someone, read a book, get started on a task, dig the garden, etc.
Lack of exercise.	Look for opportunities to exercise — walk to the shops, use stairs rather than the lift.
TV snacking; tempted by rich foods at workplace cafeteria, etc.	Avoid situations that offer excessive temptation — take a lunch from home to work, decline invitations to eat out at 'dangerous' places while building up your resistance. Either avoid any eating when watching TV, or restrict to pre-planned amounts.
Excessive caffeine intake.	Limit coffee, tea, cocoa, and soft drinks containing caffeine to five cups a day (preferably three). Consider decaffeinated coffee or herbal tea. Minimise food items and non-prescribed medications that contain caffeine, such as chocolate and cold remedies. Check the labels on food and drink purchases.
Smoking.	Enrol in a cessation programme, see a counsellor, or use a self-help book.
Excessive use of alcohol.	Reduce to the guidelines quoted earlier. If you need help, contact your medical adviser, a counsellor, or an organisation such as S.M.A.R.T. Recovery.
Drug abuse.	Stop. If you need help, see suggestions as for alcohol.

Overcoming the blocks to healthy living

People who have made the change to healthy living will usually say that it is hard at the beginning, but once better habits are developed they lose the desire to go back to the old ways. Here are suggestions to help you get over the initial hurdles.

I can't afford it

Do you see money as stopping you from eating well and following an exercise routine? Lack of finance may restrict your choices, but most forms of exercise cost little or nothing, and it is possible to eat healthily on a limited budget. See Chapter 16 for some ideas on making your money stretch further so you can achieve your goals.

Healthy eating is cost-effective. Convenience foods are pricey, and ill-health can be very expensive in terms of medical bills, time off work, or early retirement due to ill-health. Exercise does not need to cost much: walking costs nothing and aerobic exercises at home are free.

I don't have time

Poor time control can get in the way of meal preparation and exercise. Note that there are two basic truths about any activity: (1) the only way to find the time to do something is to make the time; and (2) what you spend your time on is almost always a matter of choice.

Remember that a healthy body will help you concentrate better and be more efficient, so the time spent on self-care will almost certainly be cost-effective. See Chapter 15 for advice on controlling time to achieve your goals.

Perceived lack of time was Michael's main objection to turning around his unhealthy lifestyle. However, he was eventually able to be honest with himself and admit that the stress he was feeling had already degraded his work performance and lowered his output. He was then able to see that taking some time away from work to improve his health would actually be cost-effective in the long run.

I can't do it on my own

If you find it hard to get motivated to make changes on your own, it may help to enlist support from other people. Are there friends with whom you could go walking or attend the gym? It may also help to tell others of your programme — knowing that they know may increase your determination to see it through.

If those you live with will be affected by your programme for dietary change, educate them as to why this is important for you. Are they happy to join you in the programme? If not, you may need to negotiate some compromises.

Chapters 13 and 14 contain some suggestions you may find helpful for getting support and cooperation from others.

I might feel bad about myself

Self-image disturbance, described earlier (page 36) can get in the way of change. If you fear what others may think if you go out jogging or appear at the gym in your leotards, you will be tempted to avoid getting started. If you tend to put yourself down when you slip up, then if you miss an exercise session or eat a 'forbidden' food you may end up telling yourself that because you blew it, you are obviously 'incapable' so you may as well give up completely.

Underlying such blocks will be core beliefs like: 'I need to be respected by everyone significant to me, and must avoid disapproval from any source' and 'To feel OK about myself I must achieve and succeed at whatever I do and make no mistakes.' The solution to the self-image problem is to develop *self-acceptance*. Basically, this involves separating what others think, or your own actions, from what you are as a person. Granted, this is easier said than done, but it is worth learning how. See page 80 for some help with this. Putting self-acceptance into practice might involve behaviours such as the following:

- Use *exposure* (page 87) to help you with your fears of what others will think. Deliberately go power-walking at times and in places where you know you will be seen. Wear your exercise gear when other people are around. Prepare yourself in advance with *imagery* or a *rational belief card.*

- Don't eat, drink or use drugs out of fear that others will put you down if you don't.

- Don't go on a diet simply because of how you think you look — do it for your health's sake.

- Accept that at age 50, you can't be Miss World or Mr Universe — and that's OK.

- Accept there may be weight gain when nicotine stops suppressing your appetite and poisoning your body.

- Expect to lapse. When you do, instead of condemning yourself as a hopeless case and giving up altogether, use it as an opportunity to learn and further develop your coping skills. Then get back to your self-help programme.

- If you are prone to feeling guilty about putting yourself first, remember that the other people in your life are going to be better off if you look after yourself properly. As you design and practise a more healthy lifestyle, keep in mind the wishes of those around you; but make sure you keep your own health in its true priority — right near the top of the list.

I don't feel like it

Probably the most common reason people give up on exercise and healthy eating regimes is *low tolerance for frustration and discomfort*, involving beliefs like those in the left-hand column below. On the right are some rational alternatives.

Health-defeating beliefs	Motivating beliefs
When I feel bad, I have to make myself feel better by ... (eating, smoking, drinking, etc).	There are other ways to make myself feel better — going for a run, analysing my thoughts, telephoning a friend — that don't harm me in the long run.
I can't stand how I feel when I go without ... (sugar, salt, a cigarette, etc).	I don't like how I feel when I resist the quick fix, but I can (and obviously do!) stand it. The pain is only short term (but the gain of tolerating it is long term).
It is too hard to ... (leave that cake alone, resist asking a colleague for a cigarette, etc).	It is difficult, not impossible. And I can make it easier by learning and using some coping skills.
Getting myself healthy should be easy and not require time and energy from me.	Where is it written that everything should be easy? Don't they say 'No gain without pain'?
I must feel like doing something before I can do it.	I don't have to 'feel' like it to do something! All I need is a good reason to do it — like staying healthy.

Expect to be uncomfortable as you change your eating patterns and get down to exercising. Anticipating discomfort makes it easier to cope with. Remind yourself that you will come to like new food only after you have eaten it for a while, and will enjoy exercising when your body begins to adjust. And don't view the present discomfort of moderating your diet and increasing your exercise as just a pain. See it as helping you achieve long-term pleasure and enjoyment.

The key to overcoming low discomfort tolerance is a combination of changing self-defeating beliefs, as demonstrated above, and some behavioural strategies like the following:

- Use rewards and punishments. When you achieve specific objectives, reward yourself. If you slip up, deprive yourself of some enjoyable food, drink or activity for that day. Don't carry punishment to extremes, and make it directly related to the omission concerned. Emphasise reward more than punishment. Healthy eating and exercising will eventually become its own reward — before long you will not want to miss your daily walk or go back to fat-filled food. But while your body is adjusting, give your motivation all the help it can get.

- Make it easier to resist temptation. Don't store unhealthy foods at home. Avoid shopping when you are hungry. Always have a shopping list and stick to it. Don't prepare more food than you need. Be clear about your rules: no snacking, trim the fat off meat, eat fruit instead of sweets, and so on. Do a *benefits calculation* (page 78) on smoking, bingeing or other unhealthy behaviours.

- Instead of overeating, drinking, smoking, or using drugs to feel better, work at increasing your tolerance for bad feelings. Use *paradoxical behaviour* (page 88). Make yourself do things you don't 'feel like' doing: resist the temptation to eat unhealthy foods until the desire gets out of your system; persevere with healthy food until you come to like it; keep making yourself exercise until you begin to enjoy the exercise itself.

- To stay motivated, make sure you develop a diet

or exercise regime that suits you. What happens to be trendy or to suit most people will not work for everyone. You may need to try out some different approaches before you discover what works for you.

Take responsibility for yourself. Don't blame others or the world because you are unhealthy. Get moving and take charge of your own health.

Practise the principle of *moderation* (page 62). 'All-or-nothing' radical approaches to new diets or exercise programmes usually lead to giving up altogether when things don't happen fast enough. Keep your expectations realistic — years of ingrained bad habits will not be undone in a few months.

Finally, stay flexible. Avoid black-and-white thinking over your diet or exercise routine. Don't make a pain out of what can be a pleasure. Allow yourself an indulgence now and then, without feeling guilty. When you slip back, resist any 'all-or-nothing' thinking; instead, pick yourself up, analyse the lessons, and get back on track.

Flexibility was a principle that worked well for Michael. It enabled him to become less wrapped-up in his work and get some balance back into his life. It helped him develop a diet that still allowed for some caffeine and sugar in moderation. Flexibility encouraged him to avoid the demand for an 'all-or-nothing' approach that might have set him up for failure, and instead develop a progressive programme that enabled him, step-by-step, to regain control over his health and his life.

10

Tension:
to take control, let go

When the body gears up for action, the heart beats faster, breathing speeds up and the muscles tense. These reactions are designed to meet the *physical* demands of a situation — that is, to either fight off danger or run from it.

Unfortunately, the body often gets it wrong. Most modern-day problems do not require a physical response. If a child is whining, you need to use your head not your fists. Running away when the boss criticises you may say a lot for your physical fitness, but not much for your future as an executive.

What we need to do instead is to let go, or 'relax' the tension. This reduces the arousal. When you relax, you slow things down and loosen up your muscles. *Relaxation training* is the term given to the procedure used to achieve this desirable state. Relatively simple to learn and practise, it can help in many ways. You may function more effectively under pressure, improve your sleep, manage anxiety, and have more control over strong emotions such as anger. It is used to help people reduce pain, cope with medical procedures, and lower blood pressure. Although it is a physiologically-based procedure, the personal control it provides can lead to increased confidence in your ability to cope.

Who will benefit from learning to relax?

You will most likely benefit from relaxation training if you experience any of the following signs and symptoms: muscles (anywhere in the body) are tense; you tend to be restless, keyed-up, easily startled; your heart pounds and blood pressure is high; you are short of breath; you experience headaches and/or migraines, trembling, nervous tics, grinding of the teeth, a frequent need to pass water, diarrhoea or constipation, indigestion, queasiness in the stomach; or you have trouble sleeping.

Behaviours that indicate relaxation training is needed include: impatience, hyperactivity, short temper; constant busy-ness to avoid feeling agitated; using tranquillisers or other drugs to calm down. Health problems that can often be helped by relaxation training include: hypertension, strokes, angina, heart attacks; chronic pain; stomach and duodenal ulcers; ulcerative colitis; irritable bowel syndrome; digestion problems; and rheumatoid arthritis.

Michael, the software engineer/team leader we met in the previous chapter, was a clear candidate for relaxation training. Whenever there was a challenging situation at work, he would experience tightness throughout his body. He was becoming edgy for much of the working day and somewhat short-tempered, which was uncharacteristic for him. When he noticed that he was feeling restless even at home, and tense when he went to bed, Michael realised that he had lost control of what his body was doing.

If you have any of the following conditions, discuss relaxation training with your health professional before proceeding: chest pains, hypertension, low blood pressure, cardiac disorder, asthma, diabetes, epilepsy, glaucoma, thyroid disorder, hypoglycaemia, narcolepsy, and diseases of the gastrointestinal tract; or if you have recently had surgery or an injury or have problems with your muscles.

Several mental health conditions also may contraindicate relaxation training. It is not usually appropriate when a person is very depressed, because of the slowing down associated with depression (an exception might be a depressive state where there is considerable agitation). If a psychosis is present, consult with an appropriate professional before proceeding.

The three principles of relaxation training

Relaxation training will be more effective when you keep in mind some basic principles. First, *relaxation is a way of taking control.* 'Letting go' of tension is the opposite of what your body is trying to do when stressed. There is a paradox here. By making the body 'let go' at your command, you are actually gaining greater control over it.

Secondly, *relaxation involves training.* It is not something a therapist does to you. It is something that you *learn* to do. And learning involves practice: rather than wait for a stressful situation to come along before you use your training, you practise so that you are proficient *before* you need to apply it.

Following on from this is the third principle: *relaxation is something you do.* You are not 'cured' when you have completed the training. You need to consciously *apply* it when you feel stressed. Certainly, the more you use it, the more automatic it will become — but this will happen only after you have used it for some time.

Three-stage relaxation training

Why bother with actually *learning* relaxation? Why not just buy a relaxation tape and run it every time you feel uptight? Unfortunately, much of our stress occurs in situations we are not able to conveniently leave in order to calm ourselves down. Michael, for example, knew that his boss was unlikely to adjourn a business meeting for half an hour so he could go back to his office and play a tape of New Age music. Your kids probably won't stop demanding your attention while you pop into the lounge for 20 minutes to listen to dolphin sounds.

Michael, like most people in modern society, needed to be able to stop feeling uptight quickly, in the stressful situation itself, and when other people were around. He found the solution in the method outlined here, which combines several different approaches into a three-stage procedure for achieving this goal. The many hundreds of people to whom I have taught the method have reported major improvements in their stress symptoms. It is adapted from the method outlined by Goldfried and Davison.[1]

The training will benefit you as a whole. Once you know how to make your muscles relax, regulate your breathing and focus your consciousness, you will be able to slow down both body and mind.

Introducing the three stages

Stage I is designed to help you make a clear distinction between tension and relaxation. Taking each of the main muscle groups in turn, you first tighten your muscles and concentrate on the exaggerated feeling of tension, then let go and focus on the contrasting feeling of relaxation. This takes about 30 minutes. You practise this once a day for seven to 10 days. The purpose of this stage is solely to prepare you for the next one.

In *Stage II*, you relax the same muscle groups but without tensing them first. This takes about 15 minutes. Again you practise each day for seven to 10 days. As with the previous stage, the purpose of this one is simply to prepare you for the next stage.

Stage III shows you how to relax the whole body all at once — and keep it relaxed even when you are carrying out day-to-day tasks. This is the ultimate aim of the whole process and takes about 10 minutes to complete.

The main training period will take around three weeks to complete in total. Then you will practise several simple exercises for a few minutes each day for a month or so, to consolidate the skill. After that, you will not need to do any exercises again. You will know how to relax more or less instantly in any situation. It is then just a matter of frequently reminding yourself to actually use what you have learned.

Some important things to keep in mind

You are about to learn a new skill, like driving a car or playing a musical instrument. Don't expect to achieve deep levels of relaxation right away. As you practise, you will get better results.

Adopt the attitude of 'going with' the process. You don't have to strive to relax: what you need to do is to 'let it happen'.

If you have problems with your knees, back or any other joints, don't strain them when doing the exercises. If you wear contact lenses, take them out. When you tense a muscle, you don't need to tense it as hard as you can go — that can hurt. Just tense it to about three-quarters of the maximum possible tension.

When you let the tension go, release it instantly, and enjoy the sudden feeling of looseness.

Finally, do not attempt to use the training procedure while you are driving, operating machinery, or in any other situation which requires alertness or concentration. Do your practice when you are alone, in a quiet place, and temporarily away from your responsibilities, and it is safe to relax.

Getting started

The remainder of this chapter contains detailed instructions for teaching yourself the procedure. (If you prefer, you can obtain a professionally-prepared recording of the Three Stage Method with an instruction booklet — details are given at the end of the chapter.)

The only equipment you need is a high-backed chair that fully supports your body, a quiet place, and a pencil and paper to record your progress. At each practice session, record the date, how tense you felt before you started, and how tense you were after you had practised. Use this rating scale:

Completely relaxed				Moderate tension				Maximum tension		
0	10	20	30	40	50	60	70	80	90	100

Stage I

Draw up a form with headings like the example below, then record the date and your current tension rating. The example is from Michael's practice sessions.

Date	Rating		Any comments
	Before	After	(eg, interruptions, worrying, illness, headache, tiredness, etc)
25 Sept	70	40	Had difficult day at work, slight headache
26 Sept	65	40	
27 Sept	65	35	Phone rang during practice
28 Sept	60	30	

When you are comfortably settled in your chair, check that you are breathing correctly. Place one hand on your stomach and the other on your chest. Begin breathing deeply and slowly (but comfortably). The hand on your abdomen should rise as you breathe in, but the hand on your chest should stay still. Do this for a minute or two until you feel that you are breathing comfortably (you can then let your hands rest on the arms of the chair).

You are now ready to begin working on the main muscle groups of your body. Follow these steps for each group:

1 Tense the muscles.

2 Hold the tension for five seconds and study it.

3 Release the tension.

4 Study the feeling of relaxation for five seconds.

5 Repeat steps 1–4.

6 Check that you are breathing correctly, and wait for another 10 seconds.

7 Move on to the next group.

Working through all the main muscle groups in this way will take about 30 minutes. Start with the following sequence:

1 Clench your *left fist*. Hold it tight and feel the tension in your hand and in your forearm. Keep it clenched and study the tension, hold it, study it ... (*hold for five seconds*).

2 And now let go. Relax your left hand and let it rest on the arm of the chair. Let your fingers spread out, relaxed, and note the difference between the tension you created before and the relaxation you can feel now ... (*five-second pause*).

3 Repeat steps 1 and 2.

4 Keep breathing deeply, taking the air right down into your abdomen; breathing deeply, slowly, naturally and very comfortably ... (*do this for five seconds*).

Repeat this *tense* ➤ *relax* ➤ *tense* ➤ *relax* ➤ *check breathing* sequence with the following muscle groups:

1 The muscles in the right hand.

2 The muscles in the backs of your hands (stretch both arms out in front of you and bend the hands back at the wrists so that your fingers point toward the ceiling).

3 Your biceps, the muscles in the upper arm (close your hands into fists, bend your elbows and bring your fists up toward your shoulders).

4 The muscles in your forehead (wrinkle your forehead by raising your eyebrows as high as you can).

5 The muscles around your eyes (close your eyes very tightly, creating tension in your eyes and in your cheeks).

6 Your jaws (bite your teeth together hard, and study the tension throughout the jaw area).

7 Your mouth (press your lips together hard, and at the same time press your tongue against the roof of your mouth. Feel the tension all around the mouth area).

8 Your neck muscles (press your head back as far as you can against the chair, until you can feel the tension in the back of your neck and upper back).

9 Your neck muscles again. (This time move your head forward and press your chin into your chest, almost as hard as it will go. Feel the tension, mainly in the front of your neck.)

10 Your shoulders (shrug them as though you were trying to touch your ears).

11 The muscles around your shoulder blades (push your shoulders back as though you were trying to touch them together).

12 The muscles in your back. (Leave the top of your back on the chair, and arch the middle of your back right out, making your lower back quite hollow. Feel the tension all along your back.)

13 The muscles in your chest. (Take a deep breath, filling your lungs, and hold it. Feel your chest muscles tensing.)

14 Your stomach muscles (pull your stomach in and make it very hard and tight).

15 The muscles in your bottom (pull your buttocks together).

16 Your thigh and upper leg muscles (lift your legs off the floor, stretch them out and push your toes away from you until the thigh muscles become very hard).

17 Your calf muscles (lift your feet off the floor, but this time point your toes back towards your head until you can feel tension in the calf muscles).

You are almost, but not quite, finished. You have been learning how to direct your muscles to relax, and you have gained a better understanding of the difference between tension and relaxation. You can now be aware of any remaining tension in your muscles, focus on the muscle concerned, and make it relax a little further. Go back over the muscle groups you have just worked on. As you come to each group, note whether there is any tension in those muscles. If there is, then focus on those muscles and direct them to relax, to loosen.

- Relax the muscles in your feet, ankles and calves ... (*five-second pause*) ... shins, knees and thighs ... (*five-second pause*) ... buttocks and hips ... (*five-second pause*) ... stomach, waist, lower back ... (*five-second pause*) ... upper back, chest and shoulders ... (*five-second pause*) ... upper arms, forearms and hands, right through to your fingertips ... (*five-second pause*) ... throat and neck ... (*five-second pause*) ... jaw and face ... (*five-second pause*) ... Let all the muscles of your body relax, more and more, deeper and deeper ... (*five-second pause*).

- Now, just sit quietly with your eyes closed, breathing deeply, slowly, naturally and very comfortably. For a few minutes, do nothing more than that ... (*do this for two minutes*).

- Next think of a 0–100 scale, where 0 is completely relaxed and 100 is maximum tension. Decide approximately where you are on that scale now, so you can record that score on your record sheet.

- Now have a good stretch, and be fully alert.

- Record your final score on the record sheet.

From here on:

- Carry out the same sequence each day for the next seven to 10 days, or at least until you reach a relaxation level of 30 or below on two or three consecutive days.

- Remember this is only the first step in a three-stage training process. You will not be ready to apply the relaxation skills in the outside world for a few weeks yet. Note, too, that at this stage the feeling of relaxation is unlikely to last for very long after the practice session.

Stage II

Once you have become used to identifying the difference between tension and relaxation, you are ready to move on. Stage II involves simply *letting go* each muscle group in turn (without first tensing). This will move you closer to the ultimate aim, where you are able to let your whole body relax instantly, without doing any exercises at all.

Start by recording your present level of tension on a form like the one you prepared for Stage I. Then sit comfortably, with all parts of your body supported so that there is no need for any of your muscles to be tensed.

Follow this sequence:

- Breathe deeply, taking the breath right down into your stomach; breathing deeply, slowly, naturally and very comfortably ... (*three-second pause*).

  Direct your attention to your *right hand* and let go of any tensions that might be there ... (*three-second pause*) ... Relax the muscles in your right hand as far as you are able ... (*three-second pause*) ... Just let go, further and further ... (*10-second pause*).

  Repeat this *breathing* → *relax* → *relax* sequence with the following muscle groups:

  1 Your right forearm.

  2 Your upper right arm.

  3 Your left hand.

  4 Your left forearm.

5 Your upper left arm.

6 Your shoulders.

7 Your forehead.

8 Your eyes.

9 Your cheeks.

10 Your jaws.

11 Your neck.

12 Your chest.

13 Your stomach.

14 Your hips and buttocks.

15 Your thighs.

16 Your calves.

17 Your feet.

To finish …

1 Even when you are feeling very relaxed, it is often possible to let go just a little bit more, to feel even more relaxed. To do this, count from 1 to 10, repeating the following words (or something like them). When you say each number, just let go a little bit more than before. 'One, relax, just relax …' (*three-second pause*) … 'Two, deeper and deeper, further and further relaxed …' (*three-second pause*) … 'Three, letting go, more and more, deeper and deeper …' (*three-second pause*) … 'Four, getting heavier and looser, more and more relaxed …' (*three-second pause*) … 'Five, further and further relaxed …' (*three-second pause*) … 'Six, more and more, further and further …' (*three-second pause*) … 'Seven, deeper and deeper, more and more relaxed …' (*three-second pause*) … 'Eight, letting go more and more …' (*three-second pause*) … 'Nine, your whole

body more and more relaxed, deeper and deeper ...' (*three-second pause*) ... 'Ten, just continue to relax, more and more, further and further relaxed ...' (*three-second pause*).

2 If you are now at 30 or below on the tension rating scale — that is, feeling quite relaxed — you can try an exercise that will help you relax even more. Focus your attention on the point at which your breath enters and leaves your body, and allow your body to relax a little more each time you breathe out. This will help you clear and relax your mind, as well as increase the relaxation in your body. Do this for a few minutes ... (*three-minute pause*).

3 Now decide approximately where you are on the tension rating scale.

4 Have a good stretch, and be fully alert.

5 Record your final score on the record sheet.

From here on:

- Practise this stage each day for seven to 10 days, until you are regularly achieving a relaxation level of 30 or below for about five days in a row.

Stage III

After adequate practice on Stage II, you are ready to learn how to relax your entire body inconspicuously and quickly in just about any situation, even while carrying out tasks and activities or in the presence of other people.

Your aim with Stage III is to learn how to be aware of any unnecessary tension that creeps into any of your muscle groups and quickly let it go, in a selective fashion, depending on what the situation requires of your muscles.

Follow this sequence:

1 Relax in your chair for five to 10 minutes, or until you have achieved a relaxation level of about 30 or below.

2 You need *some* tension in *some* parts of your body to carry out day-to-day activities. However, other parts of the body may not need to be tensed, and it is this unneeded tension that will be your focus with three simple exercises.

—Fix your gaze on some object on the wall, such as a picture or a light switch. Notice that to do this you need to slightly tense your neck (to keep the head upright) and your eyes (to keep them open and focussed on the object). Identify any *other* tension that has crept in (for example, in your arms, legs, stomach, etc) and let that unnecessary extra tension go, while still focussing on the object.

3 When you become relaxed again, repeat step 2 with more demanding tasks:

—hold a book in your hands and turn it over and over for a few minutes;

—stand up and look out of a window.

With each task, identify which muscles need to be tensed to carry it out, then be aware of and get rid of any unneeded tension that creeps into other parts of your body. Continue each task until you are able to remain relatively free of tension while carrying out the task.

From here on:

• Practise the Stage III exercise for a few minutes each day for several months. This will help you consolidate the relaxation habit.

Using a tape recorder

An alternative way to learn the three-stage relaxation procedure is to record the instructions for Stages I and II. Then all you have to do is follow the recording when you practise. You could record it yourself or have someone else do it for you. Speak in a slow, measured, calm manner.

An additional technique: the breathing focus

Once you have completed the three-stage training outlined above, you will be able to relax quickly and efficiently in just about any situation. There are some additional strategies you can add to your basic training. One that is particularly useful I call the *breathing focus* technique.

This procedure is good for clearing the mind when it is overactive or you are worrying and unable to relax. It can also help you get to sleep. You can use it for five minutes or so to refresh body and mind during the day. This is one of the simplest and most useful techniques I teach my clients. You have already done it to some degree if you have completed Stage II of the three-stage method above.

The technique

- Sit (or lie) in a comfortable position.

- Breathe in slowly and deeply. Take a good, deep breath right down into your stomach, filling yourself with health-giving oxygen.

- Hold your breath for about one second.

- Slowly breathe out. As you do, focus on your breath as it leaves your body. Focus on the centre of your face, visualising the breath leaving through your nose, your mouth, or both.

- Imagine that each time you breathe out, a little more of

the tension leaves your body along with your breath. Let your body — from the top of your head to the tips of your fingers and down to your feet — slump a little more each time you breathe out. Breathe right out, expelling all the old air and waste products.

- Pause for about a second before breathing in again.

Some tips to make the procedure more effective
- Maintain your focus on the centre of your face, where the breath enters and leaves your body. If your attention wanders, gently bring it back. Staying with this one point of focus will help keep your mind from drifting back to stressful thoughts.

- When thoughts intrude, simply allow them to pass by and return to focussing on your breathing.

- Whenever you become aware of noises around you, instead of trying to shut them out, focus on them briefly. Treat noise as a natural part of your environment, rather than something to be avoided. Some people find it helpful to think of themselves as 'merging' with the noise or 'absorbing' it. This strategy can be surprisingly effective when you are trying to work, relax or sleep in a noisy situation.

- Don't get obsessive about getting your breathing 'perfect'. Don't force yourself to breathe deeply. Adopt the attitude of 'allowing' it to happen.

When to use it
- Use the breathing focus technique whenever you feel stressed, especially when stressful thoughts keep intruding.

- Use it to get to sleep when your mind is overactive or your body is tense.

- Try using it routinely for five to 10 minutes one or more times a day. This will increase your alertness and concentration, and also act as a stress preventative.

I use this exercise every day, at least once (after lunch), and often again later in the day. I have a cheap kitchen timer which I set for 10 minutes to ensure I don't drift off into a deep sleep. This sets me up to be relaxed but alert, especially in the afternoon when my energy and concentration tends to be at a low ebb.

Making relaxation work in everyday life

Remember that the relaxation skills you have learned are just that — skills. They are not a 'cure'. You will benefit from what you have learned in proportion to the extent you apply it. Get into the habit of stopping at regular intervals throughout the day to consider: 'Am I tense or relaxed right now? Could I be more relaxed than I am?'

To facilitate this, develop a reminder system. Get some coloured stickers (dots or stars) and place them where you will see them through the day — on the bathroom mirror, above the kitchen sink, on the car speedometer, on your watch-strap, briefcase, purse or wallet.

Finally, keep in mind that relaxation training is not a total solution to stress. Don't neglect to deal with the self-defeating attitudes and beliefs that create stress, and which can stop you applying your new-found relaxation skills.

Overcoming the blocks to a relaxed body and mind

I don't have time

Michael could see that relaxation training would be a good idea, but was initially concerned that taking time out from work would only increase the stress he was already feeling, which would make the training counterproductive. Fortunately, on reconsideration, he realised that spending some time to develop the ability to relax his body and mind might actually be cost-effective. If he could reduce his fatigue and increase his alertness and concentration, this would increase his efficiency and productivity — which is what happened. Taking the time to learn and use relaxation, instead of resorting to quick fixes, such as caffeine or candy bars, helped him control stress more effectively in the long run. (If you have significant trouble with time, see the suggestions in Chapter 15.)

Relaxation does not seem to work

If relaxation does not seem to work for you, first check that you were ready to begin. Review the suitability criteria at the beginning of this chapter.

Have you practised the three-stage training method faithfully? Make sure you take the time to follow each step correctly, especially the daily practice. Remember, the time spent will almost certainly be cost-effective in the long run.

Your mind is actively worrying

Do some work on any worrying tendency before you attempt further relaxation training. Regular use of *rational self-analysis* is an excellent tool to chip away at this destructive habit. See Chapter 7 for detailed advice on how to combat worrying.

You become panicky

A small proportion of people who begin relaxation training paradoxically become more anxious, sometimes even panicky, when they start to relax. This is usually due to a perception of losing control as they begin to let go. Apply the principle of *discomfort tolerance* (page 164). Remind yourself that the anxiety is unpleasant but not 'horrific', uncomfortable but not 'unbearable'. Persevere through the discomfort — the sensation will pass. If you feel afraid when you close your eyes during the training, keep them open to begin with. Most importantly, uncover and deal with the thoughts creating your anxiety, using a technique such as *rational self-analysis* (page 70).

A final note ...

To make relaxation work for you, keep in mind the principle of *emotional and behavioural responsibility* (page 63). Don't blame others for the way you feel — this will stop you taking charge of yourself. Don't rely just on professionals to fix your tension — you can get advice and help, but in the end only you can put the advice into practice.

If you take personal responsibility for managing your tension, relaxation will become, as it has for Michael and many others, a valuable tool you can use in many areas of your life.

Obtaining a relaxation tape/CD

A professionally-prepared recording of the three-stage method, which includes the breathing focus technique and a printed manual, is available for purchase on either cassette tape or CD. You can obtain this package via the Internet (www.rational.org.nz/public/relaxtape.html).

Sleep:
how to make it happen

Occasionally feeling tired during the day is normal for most people. However, if this happens a lot you may feel irritable and short-tempered. It will be hard to carry out even routine tasks. Concentration, spontaneity and creativity will be affected. Chronic tiredness can increase the risk of accidents and make a person more vulnerable to depression and anxiety.

There are many possible reasons why a person may have trouble getting a good night's sleep, including environmental irritants, health difficulties, tension, worrying and unhelpful lifestyle factors. To illustrate this, let's reintroduce Denise, whom we first met in Chapter 7, and Michael, whose work-related stress has been described in the previous two chapters.

The initial cause of Denise's sleep difficulty was her long-standing tendency to worry. Mulling over problems continued even after she went to bed, and the resulting activity in her mind and the feelings of anxiety were incompatible with dropping off. Unfortunately, her sleep disturbance had gone on for so long that it had taken on a life of its own. It was now a habit for Denise to lie awake in bed at night. Consequently, the problem continued even as she successfully reduced her worrying.

Michael, by contrast, was not a worrier, but his unhealthy

diet and lack of exercise, coupled with tension that continued through the night, were keeping him awake.

Fortunately, although there are many causes of sleeplessness, there are just as many solutions! Soon we shall see what worked for Denise and Michael. If you have a sleep problem, there is almost certainly an answer to it for you.

Analyse your sleep problem

The first step is to carefully analyse the nature of your difficulty. There are two stages to this examination. The first is to keep a 'sleep log' (page 358) for about a week, then complete the Sleep Questionnaire (page 360). These two assessment tools will help you clarify your current sleep 'baseline', give you detailed information about your sleeping patterns, and identify specific aspects of your environment, health and lifestyle that may contribute to a sleep problem. Note that while you will need to complete the questionnaire only once, you can continue to use the sleep log to monitor your progress for as long as you are working on the problem.

Analysing your answers

Once you have used the log and questionnaire to identify the problem areas to work on, it is time to develop your action plan. While solutions are covered in various parts of this chapter, here are some remedies for specific items you may have ticked on the questionnaire:

- *Substances.* If you ticked any of the medications, see your doctor. Other items in this section require that you either modify your intake or give up entirely. Be wary of any use of caffeine within six hours of bedtime, or more than one standard drink of alcohol after your evening meal (note, however, that caffeine and alcohol at night do not affect everyone the same way, so you may need to experiment). Michael was surprised, when he counted them up, to discover that he was drinking about 20 cups of coffee per day. In addition, he was hyping himself up with sugar-laden candy bars he could purchase from a machine at his workplace.

- *Emotions.* Deal with any items you ticked using the strategies of *rational effectiveness training* (Chapter 6) or seek professional help if necessary. Denise identified her anxious worrying as a significant problem.

- *Physical health.* Seek appropriate medical advice for any of the problems in this section.

- *Miscellaneous.* The items listed in this section all warrant seeking medical advice. Snoring, for example, inhibits the brain from entering a key phase of sleep and reduces the body's oxygen levels at night. It also causes daytime drowsiness. Heavy snorers may benefit from seeing an ear, nose and throat specialist, as medical procedures are now available to correct the abnormalities which cause snoring.

- *Self-defeating thinking.* Finally, look at any items in the Beliefs section that you scored at 4 or 5. All the statements listed are either myths or irrational beliefs about sleeping.

    —You may have noticed that worrying about sleep makes it more likely you won't get to sleep! A vicious circle is set up. Demanding that you sleep will, paradoxically, keep you awake. Getting to sleep involves 'letting go', so trying too hard makes it less likely you will drop off. 'I *need* eight hours sleep' leads to anxiety; anxiety leads to sleeplessness; and so it goes around. This was an issue for Denise, who as bedtime approached was tending to worry about not getting to sleep — which served to keep her awake!

—Exaggerating and awfulising can lead to self-fulfilling prophecies. If you tell yourself you are going to have a bad day, you are likely to make yourself have one.

—Many people make the assumption that disturbed sleep is inevitable with increasing age. Some older people find it harder to sleep due to reduced melatonin levels; however, research shows that appropriate treatment can usually help older people sleep well.[1]

—At the end of this chapter there is an additional listing of self-defeating beliefs about sleep, with a rational alternative for each.

Some facts about sleep

Most people seem to benefit from between six and 10 hours sleep a night, with the average being about seven and a half. As you get older, sleep requirements may reduce. What matters is not how many hours you spend in bed, but rather how you feel in the morning.

It is possible to 'catch up' on lost sleep. If you miss a night or even two, one good night's rest is usually enough to make up the deficit.

There are a number of sleep stages one goes through during the night. Each of these is important, and probably serves a specific function in restoring body and mind. For example, the stage known as Rapid Eye Movement or REM sleep (so-called because the eyes are moving rapidly under the eyelids during this time) is associated with dreaming and an accelerated flow of blood through the brain. One theory has it that this stage restores the brain. The other main stage of sleep, referred to as non-REM or 'quiet' sleep, may serve to restore the body.

Get the basics right

Whatever your type of sleep problem, the first step to resolving it is to ensure that you are observing some basic, day-to-day habits that are important to good sleep. (These are referred to in the professional literature by the quaint title of 'sleep hygiene'.) Later we will look at some specific solutions to particular sleep problems.

What you do while you're awake affects how you sleep

- *Keep daytime stress under control.* Use the strategies in this book to problem-solve on things you worry about, manage time effectively, take regular exercise, and deal with emotions like anger and anxiety.

- *Practise good eating habits.* Eat sleep-enhancing foods, such as milk, eggs, meat, nuts, fish, cheese and soybeans. Have at least one hot meal each day and eat in a relaxed way, sitting down, at regular times. Avoid a heavy meal too close to bedtime.

- *Exercise regularly during the day* (but avoid exercise too close to bedtime).

- *Is it wise to nap during the day?* For some people, daytime napping makes it hard to sleep at night. But for others, napping will help them sleep better (as well as refreshing them during the day). You may need to experiment. The breathing-focus relaxation technique (page 181 is one way to refresh yourself during the day without going to sleep for too long.

Michael found that as he changed his eating habits and exercised more, he began to feel generally better in himself, and less likely to alternate between the highs and lows that resulted from his excessive intake of caffeine and sugar.

Ensure your environment is conducive to sleep

Is your bed comfortable? Keep the bedroom at a moderate temperature — not too warm, not too cool. Try to make the bedroom reasonably dark, but with provision for light to get in when morning comes. Dark and light are perceived by the brain as cues for the body system to put itself to sleep and wake up again.

Have regular sleeping hours

You will sleep better if your system becomes used to a regular routine:

- *Retire and get up at roughly the same time* each night and morning. Sleeping-in is not a good idea. Maintain your routine to within an hour every day.

- *Resist the temptation to stay in bed when you are not fully asleep.* Dozing in the morning, for instance, will make it harder to get a deep sleep the following night.

Develop a good pre-bedtime routine

- *Things to avoid close to bedtime* include vigorous exercise late in the evening (it will stimulate you when you need to be winding down), falling asleep in front of the television, caffeine, alcohol, smoking, chocolate and some cheeses. Not everyone is affected in the same way by these things — experiment to see what makes a difference to you.

- *Prepare yourself physically.* Try to be more physically than mentally tired at bedtime. Take a light walk, then a warm bath. Eat a sleep-inducing supper of such foods as cereal with milk, bread and honey, a warm milk drink, or herbal tea.

- *Prepare yourself mentally.* Avoid trying to deal with stressful issues that can't be resolved before bedtime: arguments, unhappy thoughts, anger, trying to solve problems late in the evening. To get rid of any excitement, engage in winding-down activities for about an hour.

- *Have a pre-bedtime ritual.* This will help cue your mind to begin thinking 'sleep'. For example: lock up the house, have a hot bath, get some supper, brush your teeth, change into your nightclothes, set the alarm clock, turn off the lights.

When you are in bed

- *Use the bed only for sex and sleep.* Avoid reading, watching television, or working in bed. Activities like these tend to create a connection in the brain between bed and being awake. (Some people are an exception to this rule, so experiment.)

- *Relax your body.* Physical tension is a common block to sleep. Relaxation training (see the previous chapter) can help you 'let go'. This made a big difference to Michael, who found that using the technique during the day made it relatively easy for him to apply it in bed at night.

- *Slow down your mind.* It will be hard to get to sleep when your mind is active, especially if you are worrying. The breathing-focus relaxation technique (page 181) can help. Choose to postpone problems — if you worry that you might forget them, reassure yourself by writing them down. (If worrying is a significant problem, you will find help with this in Chapter 7.) Denise did not suffer from the same degree of physical tension as Michael did; rather it was her mind that was overactive, due to worrying. As she became more proficient at using anti-worry strategies, she was able to let go of her obsessive thinking while in bed.

- *If you can't sleep, get up.* If you wake during the night, try letting yourself fall asleep again. If you are still awake after 15 minutes, get up (see page 194 for suggestions on what to do while you are up).

When you get up in the morning

What you tell yourself about your night's sleep immediately on rising can have a major effect on how you feel during the day. If you think that you 'hardly slept a wink' so you are 'going to feel lousy all day', you will probably create a self-fulfilling prophecy. Suppose, however, you think: 'Well, I have not slept as well as I would have liked — but I have got some rest. If I give myself a push and get moving now, I will most likely perk up and get through the day OK.' This self-fulfilling prophecy will do you a lot more good.

Dealing with particular sleep problems

Once you have rectified any problems of basic sleep hygiene, you may find that this is all you need to sleep well again. If, however, you continue to have trouble sleeping, scan the headings that follow to identify the type of problem that may be involved, then read about what you can do to overcome it.

You have trouble falling asleep

If it takes a long time to fall asleep, there are a number of things you can do that may help — experiment until you find the right combination that works for you.

- During the day, don't nap (unless experimentation tells you otherwise) or take stimulants.

- Two to four hours before going to bed, have a meal high in complex carbohydrates — cakes, jam, ice-cream, fruit pie, dates, figs, breakfast cereal, bread, milk, chocolate, potatoes, spaghetti, and the like.

- Don't go to bed until you are ready for sleep — tired, relaxed and calm.

- If you feel tense in bed, use a relaxation strategy (see the previous chapter).

- When in bed, say to yourself: 'I am tired and ready to go to sleep.' When you notice disconnected thoughts or muscle twitching, think: 'I am falling asleep.'

- If you are still awake after about 15 minutes, get up and follow the suggestions under the next heading.

- Finally, don't sleep late in the morning — including at weekends.

You tend to lie awake in bed

If you have had trouble sleeping for some time, your mind will have come to associate being in bed with being awake. You need to break this unhelpful association.

- If you find yourself staying awake at any time during the night for more than about 15 minutes, *don't lie in bed — get up*. Go into another room. Stay up for as long as you feel necessary, usually about 20 to 30 minutes. When you feel tired, go back to bed.

- While you are up, here are some things to do:
  —Read something boring.
  —Have some herb tea, a milky drink, a bread and honey sandwich, or cereal with milk.

—Do something physically tiring: ironing, cleaning, sorting out.

—Do crossword puzzles, logic exercises, anything that requires the brain to work in short, sharp bursts (but don't read an exciting book that will leave you wondering what happens next).

• Repeat this process as often as you need to during the night, and for as many nights as it takes for the wakefulness habit to be replaced.

Denise needed to use this strategy, as her sleep problem had continued for so long that it had taken on a life of its own. When she went to bed, her mind, instead of thinking 'time for sleep' thought 'time to stay awake and worry'. She began by using anti-worry strategies (for example, she kept a notebook and pen on her bedside table and recorded any things she was worrying about, whereupon she could tell herself that they would not be forgotten and she would deal with them the next day). Then she began to get up whenever she was unable to sleep. The first few nights, she got up about half a dozen times. This began to reduce in frequency until after a few weeks she was only waking once during most nights.

Your sleep is restless
Restlessness during the night could have a number of causes: experiment with the strategies below until you find what works for you.

• Stop sleeping during the day and see if it helps.

• Exercise vigorously (but not too late — preferably before 4.00 p.m.).

• Identify and deal with any underlying anger that may be involved.

- Establish a good pre-bedtime routine.

- Immediately before bed have a high-carbohydrate snack.

- Get up one hour earlier than usual.

You wake early in the morning and cannot get back to sleep at all

Early morning waking is sometimes a sign of depression — see page 25 to check for this possibility. If you think that you are depressed, deal with this now: either consult your health advisor, or find out how to treat yourself (see, for example, my book *Choose to be Happy*).[2] Otherwise, here are some suggestions:

- Cut out any daytime or early evening sleeping, and don't go to bed too early.

- Avoid alcohol during the evening (in fact it may be wise to avoid alcohol, stimulants or sedatives altogether while establishing your new sleep pattern, unless any of these are required for medical reasons).

- If you are taking sleeping tablets, discuss whether you should stop doing so with your medical advisor.

- Ensure you have a good pre-bedtime routine.

- Don't go to bed until you are absolutely ready for sleep. Make yourself stay awake (but not with stimulants such as caffeine or nicotine).

You find it hard to get up in the morning

If you have trouble getting up in the morning, here are the most common causes along with their solutions:

- *Your sleep is disturbed during the night.* Identify

and rectify the causes (see other headings in this chapter).

- *Your room is too dark in the mornings.* Allow for some morning light to get in (while keeping your room reasonably dark at nights).

- *You are ingesting a lot of caffeine.* Keep your intake down, using the guidelines outlined earlier in this chapter.

- *You have been taking sleeping pills for an extended period.* Sleep medication suppresses a key phase of sleep essential to refreshing your system. See your medical advisor about stopping the pills.

- *You are consuming alcohol too close to bedtime.* This has a similar effect to using sleeping pills. See the guidelines earlier in this chapter.

- *Your sleep routine is irregular,* so your internal 'body clock' is confused. Establish a regular routine of going to bed and getting up at the same times each day.

- *You are experiencing emotional or physical stress.* Use the relevant strategies in this book to deal with the problems concerned.

Your sleep times are out of sync with the rest of the world

Going to bed late and sleeping late is usually a habit people get into over a period of time. To break it, you need to reverse the process, step-by-step. Set your alarm to get up 15 minutes earlier on the first day. That evening, go to bed 15 minutes earlier. Every few days, bring your alarm and your bedtime forward until your hours are back to normal.

You can also do this the other way round. Progressively *delay* your bedtime so that you go to bed three hours later, until you eventually work your way around the clock. This will obviously require some reorganisation of your lifestyle, but it works better for some people.

Once you have reset your internal clock, keep to a regular routine.

There is noise when you are trying to sleep

Many people (not all, interestingly) find it hard to sleep in a noisy environment. Strategies fall under two main headings: reducing the amount of noise that reaches your ears, or training yourself to ignore it.

- *Reduce the noise if possible.* Install double-glazing, negotiate with neighbours about their stereos or parties, use the noise control officer if all else has failed.

- *Try to isolate yourself from the noise.* Insert earplugs or try a 'white noise generator' (an electronic device that blankets other noises in the room).

- *Use psychological coping strategies.* If you change what you tell yourself about noise, you will tolerate it better. Especially, identify any anger that keeps you awake. People can sleep despite high levels of noise (children and young people are often not bothered by it).

- *Distract yourself from the noise.* The breathing-focus relaxation technique (page 181) can help you do this. There is also a strategy I call 'absorbing'. I dislike noise, and have tended in the past to get angry, regarding it as something that 'shouldn't be there'. Unfortunately, demanding that the noise not be there fixated my attention on it! Now I allow myself to be aware of the noise, then visualise myself 'absorbing' it rather than trying to reject it. This makes the paradox work in the opposite direction. By accepting noise, it becomes less bothersome.

You grind your teeth

If you are constantly grinding your teeth during the night, get a dental check. Often some repairs are all that is needed. If all else fails, consult your doctor for further advice. Otherwise, try this simple behavioural technique:

- Clench your teeth firmly for about five seconds, then relax for five.

- Repeat this five or six times a day.

- Continue for about three weeks, or until the grinding stops.

Your bed partner keeps you awake

Does your bed partner snore? This mostly happens when a person sleeps on their back. Try moving them so they are on their side. Raise the head of the bed or have them sleep with several pillows. Put an object like a golf ball in a sock and sew it to the back of their nightwear. Encourage them to seek medical advice.

If your partner's teeth grind during the night, see the suggestions above. If jerking legs is a problem, consult a doctor.

You lie awake worrying

If worrying keeps you awake, see Chapter 7 for detailed guidance on how to break this pernicious habit. Here is a summary:

- Schedule a 'worry time', preferably about the same time each day, when you deliberately focus on your worries. Then postpone all worrying until that time.

- If you worry that you might forget to worry, reassure yourself by writing things down.

- Keep a pen and paper by your bedside. When you

lie awake worrying, firmly remind yourself that the middle of the night, when you are not fully awake, is the wrong time to try to solve problems. Make a note of what is on your mind, then promise yourself that you will deal with it the next day.

You experience unpleasant dreams

Probably everyone has bad dreams from time to time. It is possible, however, to increase their frequency and scariness by what you tell yourself about them — for example, that they are 'awful', 'intolerable' and 'must not happen'.

- Use a cognitive technique such as *rational self-analysis* (page 70) on your thoughts about the dreams. Begin to accept the dreams as a discomfort you can tolerate, rather than something you can't stand. If you see them for what they are (just dreams) and accept them, they will most likely reduce in frequency.

- If this doesn't work, then it may be appropriate to see your doctor to check for the possibility of a medical condition.

- Beware of using sleeping pills as a quick and easy solution. They may suppress the dreaming phase of sleep, but when you withdraw from the pills there could be a rebound effect with a resurgence of sleep dominated by bad dreams.

Jet lag

If you travel — say, from Auckland to New York — at 11.00 p.m. local time, your body thinks it is really 3.00 p.m. and not yet time for sleep. Dealing with jet lag warrants a book of its own, but here are a few tips:

- Avoid alcohol during the flight.

- Drink plenty of non-alcoholic fluids to reduce dehydration.

- If possible, arrange to arrive at your destination late in the day, and switch immediately to the new time.

- Organise a light schedule so you can take it easy for your first few days in the new time zone.

Shift work

Shift workers are highly likely to experience sleep problems. There are a few things you can do to lessen the ill-effects of shift work:

- Try to eat meals at the same time each day.

- Get four or five hours' sleep at the same time each day, no matter when this is.

- Avoid using stimulants to stay awake.

- If possible, keep to the same routine even on the days you are not working.

Ongoing use of sleeping pills

The use of sleeping pills is a controversial subject. Sleep medication will be helpful for some people under some circumstances, but the consensus at the present time is that they are usually appropriate only for short-term use.

The main problem with such medication is that the sleep it brings is unnatural. The dreaming phase is suppressed, and if this goes on too long you will suffer during the day. There is also the danger of addiction, with the consequent stress of withdrawal. Some sleep problems can be made worse by sleep medication. If you plan to use sleeping medication, it would be wise to see a doctor rather than simply purchase an over-the-counter drug.

Overcoming the blocks to managing your sleep

It's too uncomfortable

Persevering with some of the strategies in this chapter may test your motivation. Take, for example, the recommendation that you get out of bed if you wake during the night and can't get back to sleep within 15 minutes. Many people react negatively to this. It just seems 'too uncomfortable' to get up and break the pattern (especially on a cold night). This is even harder when it takes more than a few nights to fix the problem. Here are some suggestions to help beef up your motivation:

- Remind yourself that getting up (or changing other habits) is just uncomfortable (not awful or unbearable) and that facing the short-term discomfort will be in your longer-term interests.

- Similarly, resist the temptation to sleep in on weekends and holidays by noting that the short-term pleasure will disrupt your long-term sleep routine.

- When you feel tempted to use the quick fix of sleeping pills, remind yourself that getting to sleep straight away may be at the cost of longer-term sleep problems.

Denise had to do some hard work on her motivation, as it took a number of weeks of getting up during the night (in her case, during the winter) to overcome her longstanding sleep problem. She found it helpful to complete a *benefits calculation* (page 78) where she listed the advantages and disadvantages of (1) staying in bed or (2) getting up, then gave each item a weighting. She re-read her calculation each night before going to bed, and soon found she could recall the main details whenever she awoke. This reminder of the significant advantages of beating the problem made it easier to face the short-term discomfort involved.

It may not work for me

This chapter contains many potentially useful ideas. Treat them as suggestions, not directions. What works for some people, even the majority, may not work for you. Experiment to find what suits you. For example, try napping during the day if you feel like it, then try going without, and see which helps you sleep best at night.

I can't sleep unless everything at home is as I want it

Sometimes there will be things in your environment that make it hard to sleep, such as noise or an adolescent who stays out at nights. Don't let anger keep you awake. Apply the principle of *acceptance of reality* (page 65). If you can do something to change the situation, do it; if you cannot change what you dislike, you have two options. You can rail against the circumstance, tell yourself it shouldn't be happening, and stay angry and awake. Or you can tell yourself you dislike it and prefer it not to be happening — but there is no law of the universe that says it 'should' not be as it is. If you stop upsetting yourself over reality, you will significantly increase your chance of getting a good night's sleep in spite of it.

Denise and Michael faced their short-term discomfort and, by applying multiple strategies relevant to their particular difficulties, found that getting to sleep was no longer out of their control — they could make it happen.

Attitudes to sleep by

Sleep-defeating beliefs	Sleep-enhancing alternatives
I must be able to feel and function at my best every day, so I need a good night's sleep.	Demanding I be at my best every day will only make me uptight. Then I'll be less likely to perform at my best — and less able to get to sleep!

(Continued)

Sleep-defeating beliefs	*Sleep-enhancing alternatives*
There is little I can do to handle the tiredness, irritability, anxiety and poor functioning that results from poor sleep.	There is a lot I can do to deal with the consequences of not sleeping well — if I take responsibility for finding solutions and putting them into practice.
It's awful to have a sleepless night, and I can't stand the way I feel the next day.	It's uncomfortable — not a source of 'horror'! I dislike the way I feel after a poor sleep, but I can (and do) stand it.
I must get a good sleep every night.	I'm more likely to get to sleep if I stop demanding that I do.
I should be able to sleep well every night, no matter what.	It would be great to sleep well every night no matter what — but I'm a human being, not a robot that can be switched on and off.
Insomnia is ruining my ability to enjoy life and stopping me from achieving my goals.	Insomnia detracts from my well-being — but it will 'ruin' my life only if I let it.

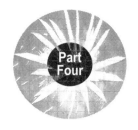

Part
Four

Control
over your life

As well as mind and body, we are also part of the wider environment
in which we live. In keeping with the bio-psycho-social approach of this
book, it is now time to turn to the final area: our external circumstances.
Control over mind and body was addressed first, because management
of ourselves is essential before we can manage the world around us.
Part Four will show how you can maximise control over a range of
circumstances, including your relationships with other people, your time,
your money, the increasing pace of change, your work, and the myriad
of smaller issues you might grapple with day-by-day.

Goals:

know where your life is going

To have control over your life you need to know where it is going — and ensure it goes in the direction you want! How clear are you about what you want to do with your life? Are you aware of your goals? Are they realistic?

Unfortunately, goal-setting is a strategy to which many people give only lip-service. It is tempting to think 'I know what I want, all I need to do is just get on with it'. Judy used to think that way. She had left school when she was 15 because she was bored and wanted money, as she put it, 'to do things'. By the time she was in her late thirties, all she had done was work in menial jobs until she got married. Her two children, to whom she had devoted her life since their father was killed in an accident when they were very young, had now left home and her life seemed empty and with no apparent purpose. She realised that very little of what had happened to her over the previous 20 or so years was the result of conscious planning.

To avoid spending your life in a succession of blind alleys, it is important to frequently check that what you *think* you want is what you really want. Explicit and challenging goals are necessary for three key reasons:

- *Goals provide motivation.* You are only likely to feel motivated to do something when you perceive that you have a good reason for doing it. The most common motivator is this: human beings, when all is said and done, want to (1) feel good and (2) avoid pain. The problem is that there are many ways to feel good. You need to know which ways work for you.

- *Goals provide direction.* Goals help you direct your life, rather than simply react to other people, events and circumstances. They provide direction to your daily activities — knowing what your ultimate aims are will help you decide how to spend your days and hours. Goals also provide direction to other stress-management strategies. To control your time effectively, for instance, you need to know what you want to achieve. Your goals will also guide your efforts to manage financial resources, maintain a healthy level of stimulation and solve problems.

- *Goals provide a sense of accomplishment.* Your achievements will be most satisfying when you can see that they result from your own efforts to achieve a clearly-defined objective. This in turn will create increased motivation to develop and aim for new goals.

Setting goals

There are many areas of life in which you will want to know where to head. Here are some of the more common:

- personal development
- intellectual development
- spiritual development
- health
- relationships
- parenting

- work
- financial
- recreational.

Judy decided that there were two main areas in which she needed to set some direction. First, she wanted to improve her health, as she felt tired and lethargic most days without any clear medical reason. Secondly, she wished to develop a satisfying career, as she was keen to work with people in some way (and believed this would benefit her personal and intellectual development, as well as addressing the areas of work and finance).

Goals, objectives and activities

Goals operate at more than one level:

- *End goals* are what you want to achieve in the long term. They are sometimes referred to as *lifetime goals* or *ultimate goals*. They are general and abstract, the things to which you ultimately aspire, the end results you want; such as, for instance, Judy's end goals: 'Keep myself healthy' and 'Have a satisfying career'. End goals may include personal, family, social, career, financial and community goals.

- *Objectives* are more specific 'sub-goals' you aim for in the medium term, such as 'Develop a healthy diet'. Objectives are designed to help you move towards your end goals.

- *Activities* are what you actually do to reach your objectives — for example, 'Restrict myself to four cups of coffee a day.'

Most people will have a small number of end goals, rather more objectives, and many activities. For each end goal there is usually more than one objective. In turn, for each objective there can be many activities. It may be easiest to visualise the relationship between these three types of goals as an upside-down tree, branching out from the ultimate goal to the objectives and then the activities — see the example in the next section.

An exercise to clarify your goals

The following exercise will help you clarify your goals and objectives, and develop some activities relevant to a high-priority aim. It is designed to draw on your 'gut feelings', so spend no more than a few minutes on each step. You can always go back later and revise your responses.

- Write a list of your *end goals* (what you want to achieve in the long term). Be honest — don't censor any of your fantasies.

- Then answer the question: 'How would I like to spend the next three years?' You may discover some new end goals to add in, and you may wish to turn some of the lifetime goals you listed into specific *objectives*. (Check: do these objectives help me move toward my end goals?)

- Now answer a third question: 'If I knew I would be dead six months from today, how would I live until then?'

- In the light of your answer, do you want to make any changes to the earlier lists?

- Now go through your list of end goals and prioritise them. Write *1* for the most important, *2* for the next, and so on.

- Select one of the top-priority end goals you would like to focus on now. Ensure you have one or more objectives designed to help you move towards that goal. Again, prioritise the objectives.

- Take objective No. 1 and list some activities that will help you achieve it. Be imaginative, write fast — brainstorm — and don't censor any ideas at this stage. Remember not to confuse goals or objectives with activities. A goal is something you want to achieve in the long run (like 'keeping healthy'). An objective is something you *aim for* in the medium term (like 'achieving aerobic fitness'). An activity is something you *do* (such as 'going for a jog each day').

- Go back over your list of activities and cull out the inappropriate or unworkable options. Then put the rest into order of priority.

- Now select one top-priority activity you can action during the next week. Decide when you are going to do it.

Here are two examples of end goals that Judy developed, with their respective objectives and tasks, to illustrate this process:

End goals	Keep myself healthy.		Have a career working with people.	
Objectives	Increase my physical fitness.	Develop a healthy diet.	Clarify what I want to do.	Get a polytechnic qualification.
Activities	1. Join aerobics club. 2. Jog each morning. 3 10 min. stretching exercises daily.	1. 4 cups coffee per day max. 2. Get healthy eating book.	1. Contact Citizens' Advice Bureau. 2. Talk to Mary about her work.	1. Get course brochure. 2. Make appointment with tutor.

From time to time, you will need to modify and refine your goals, objectives and activities to suit changing circumstances and wants. You can repeat this exercise whenever it seems appropriate.

Tips for clarifying your end goals and objectives

A key question to ask yourself when defining your goals is: 'What do I really like and dislike?' As you consider this, keep in mind the following guidelines:

- *Be specific.* Vague goals provide little direction.

- *Write them down.* This will help you be specific and fix your goals in your mind, and will enable you to review them from time to time.

- *Be honest with yourself.* If you want your goals to have motivating power, make sure they are what you really want.

- *Watch out for the 'shoulds'.* Your goals will work for you only when they reflect what you actually want rather than what you think you 'should' want.

- *Know what values are guiding your choice of goals.* Whereas goals are what we want to achieve, *values* are guidelines which affect both the goals we choose, and how we go about achieving them. 'Do to others as you would like them to do to you' or 'It is a good thing to help others' are examples of values. Articulating your values will enable you to check them out to ensure they are yours, not someone else's, and that they are relevant to you at this time in your life. This awareness will also help you develop goals and objectives that are consistent with your values. There are some suggestions for clarifying your values in the next section.

- *Ensure your goals are achievable.* Unrealistic goals will not truly motivate you — because deep down you know they cannot be reached. Set goals that can be achieved, even though they may require time and hard work. Judy, for example, wanted to work in the health field and initially wondered about becoming a doctor. She soon realised, however, that the financial cost of medical training would be unrealistic for her. After making enquiries about other options, she decided to explore three: training to become a nurse, a physiotherapist or an occupational therapist.

- *When you are unsure.* Some goals may be outside your awareness. Try taking note of your everyday actions. Ask yourself: 'What am I really aiming for by doing this? What values are guiding my choice of actions in this situation?' You may need to get into action before you can identify what some of your goals are. Try out different activities to see what you like doing. This may involve some *risk-taking* or *paradoxical behaviour* (see page 88). Judy observed that over time, she had enjoyed helping out neighbours and friends, especially when they were experiencing health problems. She concluded from this that she did possess a value about helping others, and that this could be expressed most effectively through working as some kind of health practitioner.

Clarifying your values

The values we hold determine, largely, the goals we choose and what we do to pursue them. There are many values that people may embrace. Common ones are behaving honestly, telling the truth, preserving life, caring, keeping promises, being consistent, protecting the environment, and the like. If you are unsure of your own values, there are some things you can do to clarify them.

Observe your behaviour

One way is to keep a values diary. Over a period of time, observe and record your responses — your desires and reactions — in a variety of situations. In each case, ask yourself what value(s) you think guided your responses. If you feel sad about someone getting sick, for example, you may conclude that you value good health or effective prevention measures. Anger about a restrictive by-law may suggest you value personal freedom or minimal intervention by external authority. Concern about an increase in burglaries may indicate that security or the sanctity of private property is important to you. Feeling good about having a weekend free to spend with your children might indicate that you place a high value on family life. (These three examples, if applied to the area of work, might suggest becoming, respectively, a health practitioner, a social worker, a police officer or a family counsellor.)

Make a checklist

List all the headings you can think of under which your values might fall, then use these headings as prompts to fill in the actual values you hold in these areas. Typical headings might be:

- family
- recreation
- social life
- personal appearance
- ageing
- health

- spirituality
- education
- work
- art
- literature
- music

- relationships
- romance
- friends
- sex
- honesty
- finance
- material possessions
- politics
- the environment
- law and justice.

Explore new values

Take opportunities to expose yourself to new values. Find out how other people see things. Read literature that will present you with new perspectives.

Note that the 12 rational principles described in Chapter 5 represent a set of values. As you study these ideas, reflect on them, debate them with yourself or others, and test them out, you will be introducing yourself to new values.

When values need changing

As you become aware of values that were previously subconscious, you may decide that some of them are less than useful to you. Weigh them up and, if need be, change them.

How do you change a value? By using the procedures of rational effectiveness training. A cognitive technique such as *rational self-analysis* will help you challenge an old value and develop a more functional alternative. Behavioural strategies like *exposure* or *acting out of character* will help you consolidate new ways of thinking.

Judy, for instance, became aware that alongside her value of helping others was linked another value — that 'you should always put others before yourself'. She identified this value as originating in childhood, from observing (and subsequently modelling from) her long-suffering mother, who always put the wants and needs of her family and other people before her own. By reflecting on her own behaviour over the past 20 years, Judy identified this value as one that she held. She was able to challenge it by studying the principle of *enlightened self-interest* (page 60) and adopt a more objective view of helping other people. That freed her up to still be concerned for others, but balance this with an appropriate concern for her own happiness.

Overcoming the blocks to a goal-directed life

Effective goal-setting may not always be a straightforward task. Below is a list of the more common obstacles, with suggestions to help you overcome them.

I don't have any choice

If you believe that your life is determined by outside forces, you will see little point in setting any direction for yourself. Don't wait for others to direct your life for you. Assess the values you learned as a child and, as Judy did, modify those that are not appropriate for you as an adult.

Challenge any idea that the direction of your life is controlled by external forces, such as fate or luck, over which you have no influence. While you cannot have control over all that happens in your life, you do create your own reactions. Accordingly, remind yourself that you can survive emotionally even when your plans don't work out.

I need to be absolutely certain I am choosing the right goals

Do you fear commitment? Are you unwilling to settle for one option, which means letting go of the others? Do you demand certainty and worry about making 'wrong' choices? Underlying these anxieties will be *self-image anxiety* — fear of disapproval from others and of feeling bad about yourself (see page 36) — or *discomfort anxiety* — fear of frustration and discomfort (page 38).

Remember that making mistakes does not show that you are 'useless' — all it shows is that you are a person who sometimes makes mistakes. Failure to reach a goal or objective does not make *you* a failure.

Accept that you may not reach some goals, or your attempts may have unwanted consequences. But remind yourself that risk-taking is essential to movement. Get rid of the demand for certainty and accept that the only real guarantee in life is that there are no guarantees. Remind yourself that you will survive should you set goals which you later fail to reach. Likewise, learn to see that giving away some options when you make a choice is frustrating — not devastating.

Accept that experiencing discomfort as you aim for your goals, and being frustrated when some are not achieved, are unavoidable realities of life — and while you may *prefer* discomfort or frustration not to happen, there is no law of the universe that says they 'should' or 'must' not exist.

Avoid unrealistic goals which set you up for failure — but extend yourself to your limits. Be guided by your goals and objectives — but not controlled by them. Adapt your goals in response to changes in your environment and in yourself.

I have trouble seeing that other people matter
Self-centredness ignores the reality that if we want to meet our own interests we had better take into account the interests of others. Develop the principle of *enlightened self-interest* (page 60).

To achieve satisfaction, ensure that your goals are truly your own, not someone else's; but keep in mind that you are more likely to achieve your goals if you take into account those of other people around you.

I can't seem to balance short-term with long-term gain

Some people constantly pursue short-term gains at the expense of longer-term goals. At the opposite extreme, others constantly strive towards future goals but rarely get to enjoy anything in the present.

You need two types of goals and objectives. Short-term goals bring early satisfaction. Long-term goals involve work, patience and self-denial but provide greater rewards in the future. Keep the two in balance.

Invest your intellectual capital wisely. Don't squander your resources where they will have little effect on achieving your goals. Fight only the important battles in your life — and ignore the trivial ones. When, for example, the potential exists to get into conflict with others, ask yourself: 'Is this issue *really* important to me? Will fighting this battle move me towards my goals? Or would I be better to let this one go and save my resources for the things that count?'

I can't be happy unless I get everything I want

Finally, know that you can't have everything. Remember: change the things you can, accept the things you can't, and have the wisdom to know the difference. This will help you tolerate things when a goal is out of your reach, and free you up to get on with finding desirable alternatives.

I don't deserve to get what I want

Do you believe you are too 'unworthy' or 'undeserving' to pursue your own goals, or that it is 'selfish' to do so? Don't try to convince yourself that you are in fact 'worthy' (the conventional approach). Instead, get rid of any idea that you have to be deserving or worthy before you can pursue goals for yourself. Do it simply because you want to. If being 'selfish' bothers you, remember that self-interest is part of being human — and you can practise it in an enlightened manner.

If you worry over-much about what others might think of you, accept that while you dislike disapproval, what people may think of your goals or your attempts to reach them is, in most cases, less important than achieving a satisfying life.

I don't have any faith in myself

Do you have a low opinion of your own judgement? Do you doubt your ability to achieve your goals? Do you fear that you will be unable to handle your emotions if things go badly?

Know where you lack experience and what your limits are — but keep this in balance by acknowledging your assets as well. While keeping your goals realistic, be prepared to extend yourself and take some chances. Review the principle of *ability confidence* (page 58) for some more help with this.

Know that while you don't have total control over your environment, you do have control over your internal reactions. So, when things don't turn out the way you want, you can still cope with your emotional reactions.

I'm not sure what I want, and anyway, my duty is more important

Being out of touch with your underlying values will make it hard to set goals and make everyday decisions on what or what not to do. Perhaps you continue to hold values you took on board uncritically as a child and have never checked out as an adult. Further, even when you are aware of your values, if you see life in terms of 'shoulds' and 'musts', as Judy had done since she married, you are unlikely to set goals that are based on your real wants.

Get in touch with what you really want — as opposed to what you think you 'should' want. If you discover that some of your wants are inappropriate — for example, they are not in your interests or are damaging to others — you can work at changing them; but your wants are the starting point for effective goal-setting.

Judy did get in touch with what she really wanted, and she was able to balance her sense of duty with the pursuit of her own goals. She accepts that neither she nor the people important to her will ever get everything they want, but she has reached a compromise that works for her. Now practising as a trained occupational therapist, she enjoys the satisfaction of working both for others and for herself. She has taken control over the direction of her life. Is it time to review the direction of yours?

Other people:
you can't control them, but . . .

Whn it comes to our interactions with other people, most of us would like to get more of what we want and less of what we don't. However, we know that we can't control how others behave towards us. What we can do, however, is control how *we* relate to them. This is where the real power lies in our dealings with others. It involves knowing how to effectively get across to other people what we think and feel. This ability is generally referred to as 'assertiveness'.

Assertiveness is a much misunderstood term. Contrary to what many think, assertiveness is not the same as aggressiveness. You are being assertive when you ask directly and clearly for what you want. You are being aggressive when you demand that it be given. Assertiveness, while being direct, respects the other person and takes their interests into account.

Assertiveness is the process of communicating in a way that will be heard clearly by others, while respecting what they think and feel. There are three main aspects to being assertive:

1 Asking for what you want:
   —making direct requests
   —negotiating.

2 Saying 'no' to what you don't want:

  —declining inappropriate or inconvenient requests

  —communicating concerns to others and asking for changes.

3 Expressing your thoughts and feelings:

  —stating a point of view

  —expressing appreciation.

If you stand up for yourself, people are more likely to respect you and treat you accordingly. Being able to say 'no' will help you avoid putting other people's priorities ahead of your own. Getting others to change how they act towards you will mean fewer stress triggers in your life.

By acting assertively, you can avoid the resentment that builds up through holding in feelings like annoyance or irritation. Resentment often expresses itself in physical symptoms, and the build-up of emotions can eventually overflow in response to even a minor provocation. It is better, when appropriate, to assertively express feelings at an early stage.

Communicating your concerns assertively will also help you avoid aggressiveness. Expressing what you feel or want in an inappropriate manner alienates others. Being assertive rather than aggressive is more likely to win their cooperation.

Check out your own assertiveness

Before you proceed further, complete the *Assertiveness Questionnaire* which you will find in the Extras section at the back of the book. This will help you identify any tendencies to act like a 'doormat' with other people, hold in emotions, or alienate others with aggressive behaviours. Once you have identified any unassertive tendencies, the next step is to learn what you can do about them.

A primer on managing other people

There are four key requirements for effective assertiveness:

1 You know the difference between passive, aggressive and assertive behaviour.

2 You accept and respect both yourself and others.

3 You are able to think rationally before acting.

4 You possess techniques to assertively communicate what you wish others to hear.

What is assertive behaviour?

You are being *passive* when you say nothing or you are vague and unclear. You are being *aggressive* when you demand that others give what you want or attempt to force them to comply. You are being *assertive* when you communicate in a clear and direct fashion that shows respect for yourself and for the other people involved. The chart on the next page presents some examples to illustrate the three types of behaviour.

Once you have grasped the differences between doormat behaviour, aggressiveness and constructive assertiveness, you are ready to develop specific solutions to any problems you have identified in the way you handle other people.

How to express concerns

When you have concerns about the way other people are behaving, here are some strategies that will make them more likely to listen to you:

- Deal with issues as they arise. Don't let your feelings build up.

- Take responsibility for your own feelings and what you want changed. Use 'I' statements: 'I feel hurt', 'I

Passive	Assertive	Aggressive
You say 'yes' to something you don't want to do.	You say 'no', express your regret and your hope they will find another solution.	You tell them to get lost and stop being a pain in the neck.
When someone asks you out, you say you are not available that particular evening.	You gently tell the person you are flattered but don't feel the same way, so it would not be helpful to go out together.	You tell the person they are pathetic and you would never go out with anyone like them.
When seeking information, you give up when told it is inconvenient.	You politely explain why you believe you are entitled to the information, and keep repeating your request.	You abuse the other person or immediately threaten them if they do not comply.
You say nothing when an employee has done a particularly good job on a project.	You tell the employee they have done a good job and express your appreciation.	You tell the employee that you expect them do even better next time.
You let your flatmate smoke in the house even though there is a 'no-smoking' agreement.	You remind your flatmate of the agreement, then negotiate a compromise whereby they smoke on the patio outside.	You tell your flatmate she is an unthinking bitch.
An employee is regularly late for work, but you say nothing in case you 'upset' them.	You explain privately that you want him to be at work on time, or to let you know if he is delayed.	You tell him, in front of other staff, that he is obviously incapable of organising his life.
You would like to ask out a co-worker, but you just hint that such-and-such a restaurant is a good place to eat.	You approach your co-worker, say you have heard about a great restaurant, and ask if she would like to go there with you.	You say that as you have helped out with her work she should return the favour by going out with you.
You would like to express your view in a discussion, but fear the others will view it as stupid.	When there is an appropriate pause in the discussion, you say what you think.	You interrupt and tell the others their views are stupid and that yours is the only correct one.
You feel hurt about something but pretend it doesn't matter.	You say: 'I feel hurt about what you did, and would like to discuss it with you.'	You say: 'You hurt me, and you are a bastard.'

would like you to ...', rather than 'You hurt me', or 'You should ...'

- Comment on the person's *behaviour,* not their total being: instead of 'You are a selfish bastard', say 'I don't like it when you make decisions without consulting me.' And try to criticise only what can be changed.

- Be specific. Tell the person exactly what they are doing wrong. Be explicit about what you would like them to do instead.

- Don't minimise your concerns by being apologetic or down-playing their seriousness, but avoid over-generalising — 'You *always*', 'We *never*', 'It's *totally*', and the like, are almost invariably exaggerations.

- Take care with the timing. Try to raise a contentious issue only when the other person is not upset or preoccupied. Resist the temptation to launch straight in — set the scene to get a more constructive result.

How to ask for what you want

You are more likely to get a positive response when you make your requests simply, clearly and directly, so that the other person is clear about what you want. Here are some examples:

- 'I'd like information about this medication, please.'

- 'What I want most from you is a listening ear.'

- 'Would you like to go out with me?'

- 'Please let me know when you are going to be late.'

Sometimes you will have good reason to be persistent with a request. At other times it will be appropriate to take 'no' for an answer. Learn to discriminate.

Assertive people are reasonable in what they ask for and how they put it across. They sensibly evaluate when it is in their interests to persist or to desist. And they know that a willingness to compromise will often get them more of what they want in the long run.

How to say 'no' to what you don't want

If you are unsure of your reply when someone makes a request of you, ask them for information or an explanation. Don't say 'yes' until you are sure. When there is pressure to give an answer, say you will get back to them. If they can't wait, you might be better to just say 'no'.

When turning someone down, be succinct, decisive and clear with your refusal, so the other person knows where you stand. But be polite too: then you will be more likely to get your message across without ill-feeling. Here are some examples:

- 'Thanks for offering me a special deal on the deluxe model, but I will stick to the basic machine I specified.'

- 'I am flattered that you want to go out with me again, but I don't think we are suited to each other, so I will decline. But thank you anyway.'

- 'Thank you for asking me to join your committee, but it does not fit my plans. However, I wish you well in your endeavours.'

- 'I like working in a place where we all feel good about each other, but please don't hug me when we are alone in the office.'

You can choose to explain your reason for saying 'no', but you don't have to. Sometimes an explanation will be appropriate; at other times, no reason is required. Sometimes it might be better not to give a reason at all

— when, for example, you suspect the other person is likely to argue with you.

When necessary, keep repeating your position in a reasonable but firm manner until the other person gives up. Keep in mind that if you resist for a while, then give in, the other person will keep at you even longer next time.

Handling criticism

The first thing to do when criticised is: stop. Restrain yourself from doing what comes naturally, which for most people is to get defensive. Instead:

- Question your critic. Ask for more information. Get them to be specific about their concerns.

- When you are satisfied you understand what the critic is unhappy about, ask them to be clear about what they want instead.

- Acknowledge that you have heard your critic, and show that you understand their concern (even if you disagree with it).

- Explain how you see things. Don't counterattack with another criticism or condemn the other person if you think they are mistaken.

What if the critic is overdoing it? Tell them how you feel when they over-generalise about your actions or globally rate you as a person. Explain how you would like them to speak to you when they have concerns.

What if the criticism is justified? Wear it gracefully. Being able to take criticism and acknowledge shortcomings is a sign of maturity. People will respect you for that.

Some general principles for using assertive strategies

The specific strategies described above are more likely to

be effective when you observe some general principles, given below.

- Pick your time. Requests will get a better response when the other person is relaxed rather than pressured or preoccupied. Sometimes it may be wise to arrange a meeting in advance, so that both parties are prepared.

- Be specific when describing a problem and the solution you have in mind.

- Take responsibility for what you want and don't want. Say: 'I am concerned about ...' or 'I would like you to ...' rather than 'You must not ...' or 'You should ...'. Use 'I' language rather than appealing to 'universal laws' that everyone 'should' know about.

- Start with the lowest appropriate level of assertiveness, then work up to higher levels if necessary. For example: 'Thank you for asking, but I don't think it would work for us to go out together' could be followed by: 'Thank you, but no', which could in turn lead to: 'I have already said that I will not be going out with you — please do not ask again.'

- As the preceding example shows, it is sometimes necessary to be persistent. In fact, there is a technique called the 'broken record' which is commonly taught in assertiveness-training programmes. Make sure, however, that you do not carry persistence on to the point where it becomes aggressiveness.

- Be prepared to listen to the others. People are more likely to cooperate when they believe they have been heard. Sometimes, too, you will discover new information that may lead you to change your position.

- Show other people how it would be in their interests to cooperate with you. Point out the advantages of the change you want. People are more likely to change when they believe it would be in their interests to do so, rather than because someone tells them they 'should'.

- It may sometimes be necessary to show other people why it would work against their interests to not cooperate. You might, for example, point out to an adolescent that if they fail to get home by dinner time their meal will be thrown out. But use such negative reinforcement only when the positive ones don't work. And never make a threat unless you are prepared to carry it out — otherwise, you will be training others to take no notice of what you say.

- Finally, be prepared to compromise. You will usually get more of what you want when you are prepared to meet other people half-way.

A programme to increase your assertiveness

For assertiveness training to do any good, ultimately you need to 'walk the talk'. Here are some strategies to help you put the theory into practice.

Role-playing

You will find assertive behaviour easier if you practise before using it in the real world. *Role-playing* (see page 89) is a good way to do this. All you need is a trusted friend or colleague to play the part of the other person. Describe to your helper the person to whom you plan to communicate, and coach them how to react. Keep repeating the role-play until you feel you have got your approach right.

Exposure to real-life situations

When learning how to be assertive, don't wait for opportunities to happen — set them up. This planned *exposure* (see page 87) will give you more control over what happens while you are learning, and will prepare you for when situations occur unexpectedly (as they do in real life). It is usually best to carry out exposure in a graduated fashion, beginning with easier situations.

1 Start by making a list of things you could do. Here are some examples:

—*Expressing your feelings or views.* Write about an issue to your local newspaper. Each day, tell someone about an interesting thing you are doing. Put forward an idea. Ask someone to explain a view they have expressed. Speak up about something you dislike. Protest about something you disagree with.

—*Asking for what you want.* Ask a question. Ask for service. Ask someone to help with a task. Request something from a person in authority. Ask for feedback on something you have done. Invite someone to go out with you. Start a conversation with a stranger on a bus or train. Arrange with the family for them to do their own thing while you do something by yourself.

—*Saying 'no' to what you don't want.* End a phone conversation when you feel like it. Terminate a boring conversation. Decline a request you see as inconvenient or unreasonable. Talk to someone whose behaviour you dislike. Confront someone who tries to make you feel guilty. Withdraw from a commitment you have made but did not want.

2 Grade the items on your list according to how easy or difficult you think each one will be.

3 Try to action at least one item from your list each day.

—Start with the easier items, gradually moving up the list to more difficult situations.

—Prepare yourself beforehand by using *rational self-analysis* or *imagery*, to deal with any self-defeating thoughts and emotions that might get in the way.

—Reward yourself for each item you confront.

—When you slip up and act passively or aggressively, don't rate *yourself*. Instead, rate your *behaviour*: analyse the lapse to identify its cause and see how you could do better next time.

Overcoming the blocks to practising assertiveness

Many people learn assertiveness strategies, but never put them into practice or give up quickly. The reason for this waste is quite simple. They have learned how to *act* assertively, but they have not identified and changed the self-defeating *beliefs* that stopped them being assertive in the first place. They may also, as we shall see, have picked up some new self-defeating beliefs while they were learning to be assertive!

Below is a list of the most common blocks, along with strategies for overcoming them.

I have trouble deciding what to do

Do you have trouble deciding how to react when people want your time, money or body? The most likely cause is that you are not clear about your values or about what you want out of life. Know what your goals are, both short- and long-term. Then you will make better decisions about when to say 'yes' or 'no' and how far to go in pursuing your wants. See Chapter 12 for help with clarifying goals and values.

I don't deserve to get what I want

If you believe that you are not as good as other people, or worry about their opinion of you, you will hold back from saying what you think or asking for what you want. You can overcome this by adopting the principle of *self-acceptance* (page 58):

- Understand that you do not need to be 'deserving' (whatever that may mean) to justify being assertive — all you need to do is decide what is in your interests and what is possible. Ask yourself: 'Would I teach my son/daughter (or other loved one) that they can't ask for what they want or say "no" to what they don't want unless they can convince themselves they are "deserving"?'

- Remember that even when others react badly when you attempt to be assertive, or you realise you have handled a situation badly, you will still be the same person as you were before — you don't magically become 'bad' or 'stupid'.

- Use the technique of *paradoxical behaviour* (page 88). Deliberately give yourself one treat each day for a while to disprove the idea that you must be 'deserving' to have or do pleasant things. As far as possible, make these treats things you ask of other people.

It would be 'selfish' to try to get what I want

While total self-centredness will ultimately put you offside with those around you, total other-centredness will keep you living for others and denying yourself. Either way, you will end up with less of what you want. *Enlightened self-interest* (page 60) will help you get things into balance:

- If you acknowledge that you are a self-interested human being, and view that as normal and acceptable, you will be more likely to seek what you want and decline what you don't.

- At the same time, keep in mind that it will almost always be in your interests to take into account the interests of others. Seek to build an environment where people meet each other half-way and everyone gets something of what they want.

It is too uncomfortable to stand up for myself

Low discomfort tolerance may cause you to view the risks involved in behaving assertively as too much to bear.

- Dispute the thinking involved. Remind yourself that while the risk is uncomfortable and you (naturally) don't like it, it is not awful or intolerable — you can, and do, stand it. You may find it helpful to re-read the material on *tolerance for discomfort and frustration* (page 61).

- Use graduated *exposure* to increase your tolerance. For a while, carry out one new assertive action each day if possible. Start small and build up progressively from low- to high-discomfort situations.

- As you learn and practise assertive skills, remind yourself that no matter what the result, you have the ability to cope with your emotions when things don't work out.

I might upset others

Do you think that you cause other people's emotions?

Guilt will stop you acting assertively through fear of 'hurting' their feelings.

- Review the principle of *emotional and behavioural responsibility* (page 63). Get rid of the magical belief that you somehow have power over other people and can miraculously cause them to feel emotions such as hurt. Remember that other people create their own emotions the same way you create yours — by what they tell themselves.

- As well as letting others be responsible for their own emotions, take responsibility for yours. Avoid any blaming for the way things are. Instead, get on with the job of changing what can be changed.

- Re-study the principle of *self-direction* (page 63). Set your own goals and act in ways that help you achieve them, rather than live according to the goals of others. (Watch, too, that you are not choosing a particular lifestyle simply to show opposition to authority figures, such as your parents.)

I might not get what I want

Do you think that you 'should' or 'must' always have things the way you want? Low frustration tolerance will create unnecessary conflict with others. Do you believe that you 'must' act decisively each and every time your 'rights' are infringed? This could keep you constantly alert for any perceived encroachment, and compulsively asserting your rights even when it would be better to let something go.

- Remember that nothing in life is guaranteed. Asserting yourself will not always get you the results you would like. To get any desired results, however, you need to take the risk of an occasional bad reaction.

- Increase your frustration tolerance by challenging any demands that other people or the world be as you want them to be. Be prepared to ask for what you want, but without thinking that you 'must' have it.

- Resist the temptation to gain short-term relief by using aggressiveness to get what you want. Forgoing immediate satisfaction will often help you get a better deal from other people in the long run.

- Don't get obsessed with assertiveness. Avoid carrying it to the point where you are always on the lookout for situations where your 'rights' are being infringed and where you 'must' get your own way, no matter what the cost.

- Treat each situation as different. Think before you respond, rather than always saying either 'yes' or 'no'. Keep in mind, too, that assertiveness is not a cure for every problem, but is simply one way to improve the quality of your existence.

The problem of assertive 'rights'

One of the blocks to behaving assertively is, paradoxically, brought about by many assertiveness-training books and programmes themselves. In the 1960s and 1970s, the idea was promoted that there are some basic 'rights' upon which people are entitled to insist. The theory was that if people could be encouraged to believe they have these rights, they would feel more justified in acting assertively. These assertive 'rights' now have an almost religious status.

As Harold Robb has observed, however, there are some practical problems with the notion of rights.[1] People who believe they are absolutely entitled to what they want can become dogmatic. They can feel victimised when deprived. A number of people all standing up for their 'rights' can create unresolvable conflict. *Assertive paralysis* can occur when a belief in one's rights conflicts with the knowledge that nowhere are these 'rights' guaranteed. Worst of all, pushing the notion of rights leads to less emphasis on teaching people other, more valid, reasons for acting assertively.

What is the solution? It is simple. *You don't need a 'right' to act assertively!* If you want to change your mind, you can — simply because you decide to. If you don't want something, you can say 'no' — simply because you don't want it. You can ask for what you do want, simply because you want it. You don't have to fret about whether you have a 'right' to it.

There is a much better way to evaluate your wants. Instead of wondering about your rights, evaluate *what is in your interests.* Ask yourself: 'Is it in my interests, long- as well as short-term, to (change my mind/say 'no'/ask for this)?' 'Will it help me achieve my goals?' 'Will it contribute to both my immediate and my longer-term happiness?'

This is not the same as unbridled self-centredness. That would be just as bad as the rights approach. Sometimes you will decide it is in your longer-term interests to agree to things you would rather not do, or to refrain from asking for something you want. Principles such as *enlightened self-interest* (page 60) and *long-range enjoyment* (page 61) will provide human beings with more useful guidelines than the dubious and problematical notion of 'rights'.

Self-defeating versus assertive thinking

To finish this chapter on managing your dealings with other people, here is a summary of the most common beliefs that block people from acting assertively, along with a rational alternative to each.

Unassertive beliefs	Self-directed beliefs
Other people are more important than me.	Where is it written that some people are more important than others?
To be assertive is to risk discomfort, so I had better play it safe.	If I don't assert myself, I will guarantee bad results for my life in general!
You should never do anything that might make another person feel bad.	It's good to consider other people's feelings; but ultimately, human beings cause their own emotions.
You should always give other people a good reason for whatever you think, do or say.	While it may sometimes be appropriate to do so, nowhere is it written that people always have to justify what they do.
I must always be consistent, decisive and constant so that others can depend on me.	I can change my mind — simply by choosing to. It would be sensible, however, to consider how this might affect others.
You should always try to help someone who has a problem.	I can choose to help, but I don't have to find solutions to other people's problems.
You should avoid being a burden to others by asking for what you want or sharing your problems with them.	It is good for people to help each other when that help is a free choice. Other people are just as able to say 'no' if they don't wish to grant my request.
People should always act in a correct and right fashion, and it's embarrassing and shameful to make mistakes or blunders.	It is human to make mistakes. I can take responsibility for mine and still accept myself; and I can accept others when they get things wrong.
Other people should always treat me with fairness and justice.	I would certainly like the world to be fair and just — but where is it written that I 'should' be exempt from reality?
I must never reveal my stupidity by asking questions or failing to give an answer.	It is OK — and often helpful — to say 'I don't know', 'I don't understand' or 'I'd like to think about it'.
Other people must always think well of me, and it would be unbearable if they didn't.	I would prefer other people to like me; but I can stand it — and act assertively — when they don't.

(Continued)

Unassertive beliefs	Self-directed beliefs
I can get people to like and respect me if I ignore what I want and just do things to please them.	If I act like a doormat, I will get treated as one. People usually have more respect for those who know what they want and can say 'no' to what they don't.
You can't turn people down when they want things from you.	It is for me to decide what I do with what's mine. I don't have to give my property, body, time or energy when I don't wish to, or feel guilty about saying 'no'.
It's selfish to put your own wants before those of others.	Notions of 'selfishness' or 'unselfishness' just lead to guilt and manipulation. Enlightened self-interest is a far better idea, not just for me, but for everyone.

Relationships:
how to find support without losing yourself

Getting support from other people can play a significant role in reducing the effects of stress.[1] Talking about problems seems to ease emotional tension. Annoyances can be unloaded before they become big emotional issues. Putting concerns into words often clarifies them — even if the person you are talking to says little or nothing. A second opinion will often help you understand a problem more clearly. And it just seems to make a difference to know you are not alone as you face what life throws at you.

Unfortunately, though, people sometimes fail to take advantage of support as much as they could, usually through fear of getting close to others. A common fear is that of losing control over one's independence. This chapter will show how you can enjoy supportive relationships while staying in control of your life.

Where does support come from?

Support may come from a range of people. A lifetime partner, close friends, acquaintances, relatives and co-workers are common sources of support. What kind of people will you find supportive? Probably people you can trust, people who are good listeners, and who respect your competence but can be honest with you when needed. There are many places where present or potential supporters may be located, including the workplace, social clubs, church, special-interest clubs and societies, adult education classes, local neighbourhood support groups or specialised support groups.

The four levels of relating to other people

Support operates at more than one level. We tend to relate to other people on four main levels. First, there are *acquaintances* — people we know casually; we may have many of these. Then there are *friends,* varying in degrees of closeness, of whom we will have a smaller number. We may have one or two *close friendships*. At the deepest level are *intimate relationships* — for example, with a lifetime partner — if you have more than one of these, you may be adding to your stress!

Different levels of self-disclosure are appropriate for different relationship levels:

1 At the most superficial level, we disclose little about ourselves; probably only basic facts: what we do, where we are from, the things we enjoy, or some current activity.

2 At the second level, we go beyond presenting information to stating opinions and sharing our own beliefs, attitudes, values, concerns and judgements, thus exposing more of ourselves.

3 At the third level, we communicate our emotions, hopes, dreams, loves, joys and sorrows, which are more personal to us than our opinions. We tend to communicate at this level only with people we trust.

4 At the fourth and highest level, we communicate not only our opinions and emotions, but also our inner secrets. Usually, we reserve this level for a few close relationships.

Sometimes people are afraid to make new contacts due to anxiety about how much they have to reveal of themselves. As the above description of the levels of relating shows, however, you are not obliged to tell everyone everything. Nor do you have to tell any particular person very much about yourself, until you have got to know them and decided how close you want to become. Ultimately you do not *have* to expose yourself totally to anyone — not even your lifetime partner.

Contrary to what some counsellors, self-help books or devotees of encounter groups will tell you, you won't become mentally ill if you keep some things to yourself. In fact, you might be better to suppress specific natural tendencies — like, for instance, sarcasm — when you are around other people, while you work at replacing them with better ways of communicating.

Improving your relationships

Are you experiencing difficulty with relationships? If there are problems with an intimate partner, there may be many causes, including unrealistic expectations of what such a relationship can provide, insufficient commitment, and so on. You may wish to seek professional help from a relationship counselling service, or try a do-it-yourself approach, perhaps with the help of suitable literature. At the end of this chapter there is a list of books that I have found helpful to recommend in my counselling practice.

If your difficulty is that you lack confidence in how to communicate socially, the book by Don Gabor mentioned at the end of the chapter contains some useful and very practical advice.

Do you need more support? Are you lonely? Support systems will not usually come to you: you need to get moving and seek them out. Start by listing hobbies, sports and other interests you find enjoyable. Then develop a list of possible ways to make contacts with new sources of support. You could draw up and use a form such as the one below to help you structure this exercise:

Hobbies, sports and other interests I enjoy:	Possible contacts I could make for each item:
My main work activities:	Possible sources of support for each activity:

Right now, develop one specific assignment to approach a potential source of support. Each week, go through your list and approach another contact. List new contacts as you think of them.

Keep in mind that this process requires active looking. It may take a while. Only some of the many people you meet may be suitable. But the longer you keep working at it, the more you will increase your opportunities.

Overcoming the blocks to using support

If you are lacking support or experiencing difficulties with an existing relationship, you may benefit from working on your relating skills. However, skills training in itself will not do much if there are psychological blocks that stop you from effectively using such skills. Accordingly, the rest of this chapter will focus on identifying the most common blocks and showing what can be done to overcome them.

I don't think I am good enough

If you tend to engage in negative self-rating, this will show in self-defeating behaviours such as avoiding closeness, seeing yourself as undesirable and acting accordingly, or failing to look after your body and mind.

- Re-study the principle of *self-acceptance and confidence* (page 58) and the techniques you can use to put self-acceptance into practice (page 80).

- If you worry that others may reject you, remind yourself that if this were to happen you would still be the same person afterwards — *you* would not change. Acknowledge any shortcomings in your social skills that may have contributed to the rejection, so you can learn from it, but rate the *behaviour* — not *yourself*.

- Use the positive attributes you do have to attract new friends and sources of support, and believe that what you have to offer is of some value. Confidence will increase as you work at making improvements so that you will have more to offer others.

- Put these new ways of viewing yourself into practice with *exposure* (page 87) and *stepping out of character* (page 88). Confront any fear of revealing yourself to others by doing it (sensibly, of course). Ease your anxiety with *rational self-analysis* (page 70) and *imagery* (page 83).

I get too anxious in social situations

Do you become overly self-conscious in social situations, preoccupied with how you think you are coming across to other people? Do you fear being rejected or looking foolish or embarrassing yourself? Underlying these fears will, usually, be self-rating as described above, coupled with self-defeating beliefs like 'I must perform well and be seen as a competent communicator' or 'I couldn't stand to do anything that might lead to embarrassment.'

- Re-study the principle of *tolerance for discomfort* (page 61). Remind yourself that while you won't like rejection or embarrassment, it will not kill you.

- Confront your social anxiety with *exposure* (page 87). Deliberately get into social situations. Stay with the situation and the resulting discomfort. When you ride out your discomfort, you will discover that it does not kill you.

- Try *distracting* from your self-consciousness by actively listening to the person with whom you are communicating. (As well as reducing your anxiety, this will also help get you get started with building relationships.)

- Use *relaxation* techniques (see Chapter 10) on any physical tension.

- Prepare yourself in advance for social situations. Use *imagery* (page 83) — vividly imagine yourself in the situation, disputing the anxiety-creating irrational beliefs and using effective communication skills. *Role-play* new ways of communicating with someone else who will give you feedback on how you are doing (see page 89).

I'm afraid of getting close to people

Do you tend to avoid more than superficial involvement with others? The most common causes are fears of rejection, trusting others or getting hurt. Catastrophising is most likely involved: rejection is seen as *awful*; to have a confidence revealed as *catastrophic*; or to begin a relationship and then lose it as *unbearable*.

- There are three rational principles that can help here: *tolerance for frustration and discomfort* (page 61), *risk-taking* (page 62) and *acceptance of reality* (page 65).

- Learn to see rejection and the other unwanted events as unpleasant but not 'horrific', as undesirable but not 'unbearable'. Rejection and embarrassment will not kill you. You can stand it when others do not treat you as you would like or otherwise behave badly towards you.

- Relating to others is always a risky business. You will get rejected or let down from time to time. Remind yourself that the risk is worth the potential gains, and is much better than the certainty of getting no support at all by playing it safe.

- When friends and acquaintances turn out to be less than perfect human beings, and let you down and say or do hurtful things, accept they are just like you — fallible. Then you will be able to go on relating to them.

I keep getting jealous

Do you get upset when friends and acquaintances spend time with other people? Jealousy is usually based on lack of self-acceptance. You may have an internal demand that your friends always put you first — so you can be constantly reassured that, because you are the most important person to them, you must be OK. This will create anxiety for you, and jealousy will put restrictions on others that they are unlikely to tolerate for long.

- If you accept yourself, you will have little need to feel jealous about others.

- Work on directing your life in all areas (see the principle of *self-direction*, page 63). Then you will be less likely to become dependent on a particular relationship.

- Remember that your emotions are caused not by what your friends do, but rather by what you tell yourself about their actions.

- Involve yourself in hobbies and other pursuits that you find absorbing and that don't involve the people towards whom you feel jealous.

- Confront any jealousy with *exposure* (page 87): actually encourage your partner or friends to have social contacts and interests other than yourself.

I'm afraid of being lonely

Fear of being alone often leads to conformity or destructive relationships. Also, if you can't enjoy your own company it is unlikely that others will. Loneliness compounds itself.

Loneliness actually has little to do with being alone. You can feel lonely in a crowd. Loneliness results from self-defeating beliefs about being on your own — in particular, beliefs about your own 'unworthiness'. Accepting yourself will reduce any need to have other people around you to 'make you feel good'.

- Develop hobbies and interests that do not depend on other people but which you find absorbing.

- Confront loneliness with *exposure* (page 87). Get used to your own company by deliberately organising to be alone while filling your time with satisfying activities.

I'm afraid of losing my independence

Are you *overly* independent — an 'I don't need anyone' individual? If you fear getting close to others because you think you would lose your independence, there are some things you can do to reassure yourself:

- Re-study the principle of *emotional responsibility* (page 63). Remember that you, ultimately, have control over your own emotions — so you can accept support from others while being confident that whatever happens, you will still be able to cope with your feelings.

- Set and maintain appropriate boundaries which even close friends do not cross. Allow people only as far as you choose when it comes to your time, body, money and property. If you have difficulty saying 'no', see the previous chapter.

- If you make sure you are directing your own life in all respects, then when you actively seek the support of others you can be confident you will be more likely to remain your own person.

Other people keep taking from me but never give back

Do you see yourself as always giving to others, but not (apparently) taking back from them? This may be due to a difficulty in asking for what you want, in which case you will find help in the previous chapter. However, there is another, less obvious cause of this problem. I call it the 'social worker' syndrome. Are you available to help when your friends want you, but seem to expect nothing in return? Your selfless behaviour may really be for yourself. It puts you in a one-up position to the other person, enabling you to boost an otherwise poor ego. It is yet another sign that self-acceptance is lacking — you 'help' others to convince yourself you are OK. Unfortunately, your 'selflessness' adds to your stress — the unequal nature of the relationship means that you give support but don't get it in return.

- Re-study the principle of *enlightened self-interest* (page 60). Learn to see that meaningful relationships are based on mutual self-interest (reciprocity).

- If you do want to be a social worker, go and get trained, then obtain a group of clients *separate* from your friends.

People complain that I take but never give

At the other extreme, there are people who take but don't give. Do you hold demanding expectations of friends and acquaintances, expecting them (for example) to be there seven days a week for support, company, baby-sitting or whatever you want of them? Do you think they should be prepared to loan you money or do other things for you without question? Do you demand that they be willing, in the name of friendship, to take whatever you do or say to them without complaint, or be willing to sacrifice their own desires and wishes in order to fulfil yours? Eventually, people will get fed up and either withdraw their support or give it grudgingly; or, worse, slip into the 'social worker' role described above and treat you as though you were a client rather than a friend.

- Again, *enlightened self-interest* (page 60) is the key

to avoiding this problem. Give, in order to receive. Attend to others' interests, because they will be encouraged to attend to yours.

- Consider not just what others have to offer you, but what you have to offer them.

- If you want help without having to give anything in return (and sometimes this is perfectly valid), you need to see a professional counsellor.

I find it hard to respect others

Are you inclined to behave inconsiderately towards others and show intolerance of their shortcomings? Lack of respect for others usually reflects a lack of respect for oneself. Putting other people down is, most often, an attempt to boost a shaky ego.

- Re-study the principle of *self-acceptance* (page 58). If you accept yourself, you will find it easier to accept others.

- It may also be appropriate to review the principle of *long-range enjoyment* (page 61). Be able to choose, when appropriate, to forgo immediate satisfaction of your desires in order to build better relationships that will provide support in the long term. Propositioning a colleague for sex, or taking out your anger on a friend, may ease your frustration in the short term but lose you a source of support in the long term.

i tend to hide behind a front

Do you change how you talk and act according to the people you are with? The trouble with this is that no-one ever gets to know just who you are — and you may attract people with whom you are not compatible.

- Don't try to be all things to all people.

- Re-read the material on *self-knowledge* (page 58).

- If you know yourself, it will be easier to let other people get to know you as you really are. (This doesn't mean staying as you are; you may choose to improve aspects of yourself over time.)

Support or isolation?

Isolation beliefs	Rational alternatives
It would be terrible to share something of myself with others and have them turn it against me.	It would be disappointing, but hardly a source of terror! And although I wouldn't like it, I could survive it.
I must be absolutely sure that other people are trustworthy before I could open myself up to them.	It is desirable that other people be trustworthy, and I will be sensible about who I trust — but demanding an absolute guarantee will ensure that I never trust anyone.
I could not bear to let myself get close to someone and then have them reject me, so it is not worth the risk.	If I don't take the risk, then I *guarantee* isolation and lack of support. Rejection is disappointing — but hardly unbearable. After all, it has happened in the past and I am still alive!
True friends should be prepared to do things for you without expecting anything in return.	Why on earth would anyone want to relate to me (or anyone else) as a friend unless they also got something out of the relationship?
I couldn't stand the embarrassment if I made a fool of myself in front of other people.	While I dislike embarrassment, it does not kill me. Telling myself it is unbearable only makes it feel worse than it needs to.
It is unbearable to feel lonely, so I must have other people around me.	Feeling lonely is unpleasant — not 'unbearable'. And being alone is not what causes loneliness. I would be better to learn to be more comfortable with my own company.

(Continued)

Isolation beliefs	Rational alternatives
True friends are either there for you totally or they're not worth having.	Where is it written that friends should be totally committed? I can enjoy what I get from people with all levels of commitment to me.

Further reading on managing relationships and getting support

This chapter has focussed on getting support and overcoming the blocks to maintaining supportive relationships. As mentioned earlier, for the reader who wishes to go further and develop skills in social communication or find or develop a long-term relationship, there is some excellent literature available on those topics:

Burns, David. (1985). *Intimate Connections*. New York: Penguin.

Gabor, Don. (1983). *How to Start a Conversation and Make Friends*. London: Sheldon Press.

Hauck, P. (1977). *Making Marriage Work*. London: Sheldon Press.

Hauck, P. (1983). *How to Love and be Loved*. London: Sheldon Press.

Montgomery, R. & Evans, L. (1982). *Living & Loving Together: A practical step-by-step manual to help you make and keep better relationships*. Ringwood, Vic: Viking O'Neil.

15

Time:
do what's important to you

By now you will have realised that many of the strategies for maintaining effective control over your life — exercising, relaxation, recreation, and so on — require time. Unfortunately, important though it is, time control is a strategy that many people study but few practise. One reason for this is a misunderstanding as to what time control is about. Many people think it is a dry subject concerned solely with efficiency. But this is not the case. Time control is not about 'efficiency' — it is about *effectiveness*. It is about controlling time in order to achieve your goals. It is about planning and prioritising so that your time gets spent on what is really important to *you*.

Michael, the software engineer/team leader we met earlier in the book, had lost contact with what was important. His solution to stress was to put his nose to the grindstone and work his way through whatever was on his desk. He did not stop to consider better ways of using his time, because he believed that such reflection would use time he should put into actually doing the work. What this showed was that he had not yet made the transition from worker to manager.

When Michael was a software engineer, the work was allocated to him by someone else. All he had to do was keep at it until each job was finished; then he would be given the next task. After his promotion to management, all that changed. Now he had to juggle many tasks, all competing for his attention. The only time he would prioritise a task was when someone told him it was urgent. He had no conception of grading tasks according to their importance. His 'nose-to-the-grindstone' approach, while appropriate before, was now dragging him deeper into the mire of inefficiency, poor time control and increasing stress.

Not everyone with a time problem has lost control to the same degree as Michael. For many people, the issue is not so much one of excessive stress as one of failure to achieve desired goals. Theresa is a good example of someone who was managing time well enough to get by with day-to-day life, but not well enough to get working on a long-standing dream, in her case writing a book about growing up in a country town. Arriving at age 55, Theresa had begun to think that her vision would never become a reality.

Know why you want to control your time

When deciding how to use your time, there are three questions to regularly ask yourself:

1 'Where do I want to go in my life?'
2 'What is the best way to get there?'
3 'Am I going that way?'

If controlling your time is to serve any useful purpose, you need to know what you are working toward. That means being clear about your values and overall goals, and your monthly, weekly and daily objectives. A goal-oriented approach will keep you in touch with some basic principles of time control:

- What is important and what is urgent are not necessarily the same.

- The idea is to achieve your goals by working smarter — not harder.

- People who achieve their goals don't 'find' time for what is important — they *make* time.

- Effective time control will be enlightened — taking into account the aims and goals of other people is the best way to achieve your own.

Both Michael and Theresa were out of touch with the first three of these principles. Michael was responding to tasks at work that had upcoming deadlines without checking whether they were more important than other, less urgent tasks. Theresa's whole lifestyle was based around the idea that what needed doing now was what mattered most. The problem with this approach to using time is that for most people there are always things that appear to 'need' doing 'now'. For Michael, the statistics report due tomorrow took priority over spending time integrating a new team member. For Theresa, repainting the windows took priority over preparing an outline for a book that had no deadline and did not, as she told herself, 'need' to be written. Michael knew that the long-term functioning of his team was more important than the statistics report. Theresa knew that, while leaving the windows another year or two would make them more difficult to repaint, this was not critical — nor as precious to her as the book.

Do you need to improve your control of time? Check this out by completing the *Time Control Questionnaire* in the Extras section at the back of the book. Note the items on which you score more highly so that you can give them priority as you work to take control over your time. (By prioritising, you will be starting to practise good time control!)

Know what matters

The key to time control is to spend your time on what is important. So what is important? Whatever helps you achieve your goals. Take the advice of time management consultant Alan Lakien[1] and continually ask yourself 'Lakien's question': 'What is the best use of my time right now?'

This question applies to all areas of your life — recreation, family and work. Worrying about something you forgot to do at the office is a poor use of time when you are trying to relax with a book. Thinking about your next project is a poor use of time when your partner is trying to communicate about a family problem. Keep in mind that there are four categories of time usage:

1 important and urgent;

2 important but not urgent;

3 urgent but not important;

4 not important and not urgent.

Many people, like Michael and Theresa, miss the point that what is urgent is not necessarily important. The idea is to concentrate your efforts on categories (1) and (2).

Be aware, too, of the 80/20 rule: '80 per cent of the benefit comes from 20 per cent of the time and effort expended on a task. The other 20 per cent of gain takes 80 per cent of the effort and time.'[2] Use your time where it counts. Don't strive for perfection when 80 per cent would do the trick. Five 80-per-cent tasks add up to 400 — one 100-per-cent task adds up to only 100.

When she did finally start on her book, Theresa needed to challenge herself on the 80/20 rule. She realised that she was spending large amounts of time refining some portions that were already more than adequate, blocking her from getting on with the rest of the book.

Plan

Planning is one of the keys to controlling time rather than having it controlling you. Plan for next year, next month, next week, then for each day. List tasks that are aimed to achieve your objectives, and put them in order of priority.

- *Plan all significant projects* (including home and social events). List all the things that need to be done and their deadlines. Set a starting time. Estimate how much time you need, and add one-third to cover any unexpected problems. If appropriate, transfer specific items to your diary. If you have a planner-type diary or personal digital assistant (PDA), keep your project lists in it. Michael's breakthrough occurred when he started to book tasks into his electronic diary, which showed him that there was not time to do everything and that prioritising was essential.

- *Break goals and larger tasks down into manageable steps.* This will help you get started, and crossing off each completed item will show you how things are going. Writing a book is a long-term project that will often be spread over several years, so breaking the overall task down into smaller sub-tasks was essential for Theresa. She identified the major sub-tasks as: (1) prepare an outline; (2) research and collect material; (3) seek permission to use certain materials, including photographs; (4) prepare a first draft; and so on. She further broke down the outline preparation task into smaller steps: (1) learn to use the outline feature in the word-processing program; (2) choose chapter headings; (3) outline one chapter per week; and so on.

- *Prioritise tasks in terms of their importance.* Remember that important tasks are those that move you towards your predefined goals and objectives. Michael, for example, decided that team cohesion was a priority, and this guided his day-to-day decisions on such items as whether to train a new staff member or update the computer cleaning protocol.

- *Ignore things that are of low usefulness* to achieving your goals. Emphasise what you want to accomplish (the outcomes) rather than what you do (the outputs).

- *Maintain a diary* and record in it all your appointments or things to remember (both personal and work-related). Ensure you look at the diary every morning (instead of simply attending to the work that is sitting in front of you) in order to stay on track with the priorities.

- *Keep a notebook or PDA with you all the time*, in your pocket or handbag. You can then note down any items you want to recall later on.

- *Be flexible and realistic in your planning* — allow extra time for unexpected interruptions, and ensure your plans are realistic. Don't schedule more into a day than you can reasonably expect to achieve. Allow adequate time for travelling where this is necessary, so you are not driving fast in a panic, or getting stressed in the queue at a ticket counter.

How to get started — and finished

Getting started
Carry out the items on your daily list, working as follows:

- Start with the top-priority items first, then move to those further down.

- Cross off each item as you go — the sense of completion will be motivating.

- Ensure you keep breaking down larger tasks into small, manageable steps. This will make it much easier to get started than if you are confronted with a few huge and overwhelming projects.

Getting finished

Getting started is only half the story. Getting the job finished requires an ongoing focus on what is important to you, and management of the things that might distract you. For some people, there will also be the challenge to overcome perfectionism that might lead them to breach the 80/20 rule discussed earlier.

- *Keep your desk or work area uncluttered* to avoid other work distracting you. Do you prefer to keep waiting work out of sight? If so, list 'to-do' items in your diary or planner, then file everything away where you can find it at the appropriate time. Alternatively, if you are a 'visual' person who prefers to keep everything in view, organise your 'piles' into categories and use colour-coded folders.

- *Maintain a proper filing system.* Every year, clean out unneeded papers and put the rest in a box somewhere, so you work only with papers you need currently.

- *Set deadlines on specific sub-tasks.* This will help you avoid any perfectionist tendency to waste time getting a task 'just right'. One proviso, however — don't make finishing an absolute demand. Sometimes you may benefit from setting a task aside, doing something else, and coming back to it later when you are refreshed.

Creating extra time

It may well be possible to create extra time, thus enabling you to achieve your objectives faster. Here are some ways to bring this about. Mark the ones that you think are relevant to you.

Get rid of time-wasters
Get rid of any of the following that apply to you:

- Low-importance activities — for example, unnecessary paperwork or reading, tasks that don't contribute to objectives.

- Looking for things you can't find due to a poor filing system or hoarded clutter.

- Inadequate equipment — for example, slow computers, inefficient software, having to share equipment often.

- Unnecessary travel or waiting, duplication of effort, unnecessary or poorly-run meetings.

- Inadequate information — for example, unclear task requirements, people not available for discussion.

- Leaving tasks unfinished and having to re-do them from the beginning.

- Reduced speed — for example, through dreaming, fatigue or poor concentration.

- Low-priority interruptions — for example, casual telephone calls, people dropping in, distractions of a nice view or noisy environment, extended coffee breaks and idle conversation. Be prepared to tell people you are busy. Put a sign on your door when you are unavailable. (Ensure, however, that the paperwork you are making time for is more important than contact with the people you will be avoiding.)

Get the clutter out of your life
When you throw something out, you can never be certain that it will not be needed at some time in the future. If your

discomfort tolerance for uncertainty is low, you may find yourself with such a collection of clutter that a lot of your time is spent simply sorting through it trying to find the things you want. To break free from controlling clutter:

- don't get tied up in knots with protective measures such as over-documentation or unnecessary filing

- prepare and commit yourself to a plan to get rid of clutter within a set period — action that plan on a daily or weekly basis, getting rid of a bit at a time[3]

- use *rational self-analysis* (page 70) to prepare yourself emotionally to throw stuff out

- if your anxiety about getting rid of clutter is due to obsessive-compulsiveness, you may find it helpful to study the chapter on this problem in my book *Fear-Less*.[4]

Spend less time on tasks

- Give yourself deadlines and stick to them.

- Be aware of dawdling signals, such as daydreaming, reading the same words twice, talking to other people, and so on.

- Handle paperwork once: read it, decide if any action is required, then act on it or file it.

- Make lists rather than leave files lying around. This way you don't have to keep sorting through the files to find what you need.

- Where possible, finish tasks at one sitting. This will be easier when you have broken down goals and large tasks into smaller 'bite-sized' pieces which can be managed in one go.

- Regularly ask yourself Lakien's question (page 255) to check whether you are making the best use of your time.

Get rid of or avoid some tasks

- Say 'no' to requests and tasks that don't contribute to specific (and desired) objectives.

- Delegate when you can.

- Quickly scan rather than read your mail. Throw out or re-route items of low or no priority to you.

- Keep minimal records — don't file items you can refer to elsewhere, unless they have special importance to you.

- Simply wipe low-value tasks off the bottom of your to-do lists. (Are you *ever* likely to action them?)

Save time by spending money

- Buy computer software that helps you work efficiently, even if it costs more than the 'free' package that came with your computer.

- A fax machine or e-mail program may save you time that you would otherwise spend trying to catch people on the telephone.

- Would it be cost-effective to pay an out-worker to do some of your work, or a contractor to mow your lawns while you get on with tasks only you can do?

Do two things at the same time[5]

- Listen to an inspirational tape while driving. (But concentrate on the road!)

- Plan an activity while doing the housework.

- Use waiting time productively — read a file while waiting for someone to come to the telephone, take some reading with you to appointments, keep a list of quick tasks you can do whenever you are caught waiting.

- Be careful, however, not to overdo this. For example, don't plan a project while playing with your children, or have so many things on the go that you get distracted from finishing any one task.

Spend less time on some activities

- Forgo that lie-in and get up earlier in the morning.

- Watch less television: plan your viewing in advance and watch only high-priority programmes.

- Shorten time spent socialising on the telephone.

Manage yourself

Ensure that you look after yourself, so you are capable of using your time effectively. Exercise, healthy eating and time out will all improve your ability to concentrate and think clearly. It was important for Michael to change his unhealthy lifestyle, as described in an earlier chapter, to get his brain working more effectively so that he could change how he handled his work.

To stay alert during the day, drink lots of water, take regular breaks where you get up and move around, do stretching exercises, and take short naps or use brief relaxation techniques.

Do you work best in the morning, afternoon or evening? Use your biological 'prime-time' for the most important tasks or for those that require good cognitive functioning.

Avoid inefficient or unhealthy practices. Don't routinely take work home, or go to the office on weekends. Avoid overtime as much as you can: if you know you can continue with the task after hours, you will slow down during your normal working day.

A programme for moving to better time control

Identify your current problems

The first step towards improving your control of time is to find out where the time is currently going. A good way to do this is to keep a daily time-use log for a week or so. Record the following items:

- Each activity.

- The time you began the activity.

- A rating of each activity's priority in terms of how it contributes to your goals and objectives: 5 = no importance, 4 = low importance, 3 = moderate importance, 2 = high importance, 1 = top importance.

- A rating of each item's urgency: 5 = needn't be done by any particular time, 4 = get around to doing, 3 = do sometime soon, 2 = do as soon as possible, 1 = requires immediate attention.

- If it was prearranged, put a tick; an interruption, put a cross; or something you initiated but did not plan, put an asterisk.

You may find it useful to view your day as consisting of three segments: (1) waking up in the morning through to lunchtime, (2) from lunchtime through to your evening meal, (3) from your evening meal through to going to sleep. Fill in your log at the end of each segment. A sample from Michael's time-use log is given on the next page.

At the end of each day, analyse your entries and answer the following questions:

- *Did I plan my activities each day?* Were my objectives clear, the tasks listed, and priorities set for each task?

Time-use log

Time	Activity	Importance	Urgency	Prearranged	Comments
8.30	Checked voice-mail	3	2	✳	
8.35	Talked to Judith	5	5	✗	Enjoyed the chat, but too long
9.00	Team meeting	2	2	✓	Useful for communication
10.00	Jack re technical problem	2	1	✗	Could we avoid these emergencies?
10.25	Started production report	4	1	✓	Better to have started this earlier

- *Did the most important items get the most attention?* What percentage of activities were important, urgent, both, or neither? Did urgent items crowd out important items? Did I give the right amount of time to each item? Which activities deserved more time than they got?

- *What could I have done more efficiently?* Could I have done it faster, in a more simplified way, or with less detail?

- *What could I have avoided?* Could some things have been delegated, done later, or not done at all?

- *What time-wasters* (page 259) *could I try to eliminate or reduce?* (Keep a list of your own time-wasters. At the end of the log-keeping period, decide which are the most problematical and work on those.)

- *To what extent did I achieve my goals?* (This includes objectives for the day and overall life goals.) What goals appear to be neglected in my daily/weekly activities? To what extent am I putting my time into the goals that are important to me? What activities can I develop to more effectively move toward my goals?

Develop an action plan

Having identified and listed your particular time control problems, check their causes and develop a solution for each one. Start putting the solutions into practice immediately, and see how they work. Fine-tune the solutions as required.

Overcoming the blocks to time control

I stated at the beginning of this chapter that time control is, unfortunately, one of those activities that many people study yet fail to use. Here are some of the more common reasons. See which are true for you.

I can't help putting off difficult tasks

People put off difficult or unpleasant tasks for three main reasons: (1) *Low discomfort tolerance* — the short-term relief from avoiding nuisance, unpleasantness or pain can be very attractive; (2) *perfectionism* — the job has to be done perfectly or not at all; and (3) *low frustration tolerance* — they object to being told what to do, or believe they can't do anything unless they 'feel' like it (an increasing problem in our feelings-focussed world).

Theresa had been procrastinating for years. She felt uncomfortable when she considered the size and long time-scale of the task involved with writing a book. There was also some anxiety that she might not be up to the task. She worried that if she failed, she would then end up feeling bad about herself. It was easier to avoid the discomfort by thinking of more 'urgent' tasks and putting off getting started on the book until she had more time — which never seemed to happen.

To overcome procrastination:[6]

- Carry out a *rational self-analysis* (page 70) to uncover and change any self-defeating beliefs that get in the way.

- Complete a *benefits calculation* (page 78) on the short-term gain of avoidance versus the long-term gain of getting started.

- Accept that discomfort and frustration are normal, inevitable and tolerable — then you will feel more like facing the tasks you see as unpleasant, and discover that once you get started they do not seem anywhere near as bad.

- Use the technique of *paradoxical behaviour* (page 88): deliberately seek out unpleasant or worrying tasks to give yourself practice in facing them.

Theresa found that analysing her fears and preparing a benefits calculation helped her identify the discomfort and self-image issues that were blocking her, and clarify that the potential gains of writing the book (even if was never actually published) outweighed the costs to her of allocating the time required.

There are too many demands on my time

Do 'shoulds' and 'musts' distract you from your own priorities? Perhaps you believe you should put the goals of other people ahead of your own. Or you may have a 'should' about hard work or duty which leads you to think that as long as you are keeping busy, everything is all right — irrespective of how much you are achieving. A variation on this is the idea that the harder you work, the more you get done.

- Note that working smarter rather than harder usually gets more done.

- Use *rational self-analysis* (page 70) to uncover and combat any demanding beliefs that distract you from your priorities or keep you working just for the sake of work.

- Complete the *time-use log* described earlier to see which of your activities are not achieving much.

- Use *paradoxical behaviour* (page 88) to disprove the belief that you can't do anything unless you 'feel' like it. Commit yourself to deliberately do one thing each day that you don't feel like doing. Keep it up for about a month or until you think you have got the message.

Your time may be filled solving problems for others, slavishly following workplace procedures, or attending unnecessary meetings. This may result from fear of disapproval, distorted self-interest, or lack of self-direction. To help yourself:

- Use the principle of *enlightened self-interest* (page 60). Don't leave it to others to organise your time and your life — stay focussed on your own goals and objectives. At the same time, however, keep in mind that to be effective you need to take into account the goals and concerns of others. Keep the two in balance.

- Conversely, don't blame others because you fail to get everything done. You will make more progress if you see yourself as responsible for acting assertively and seeking constructive changes.

- Make a strong commitment to stick with tasks and see them through, irrespective of what others are choosing to do with their time.

- Avoid solving problems for others unnecessarily — train people, by your actions, to think for themselves.

- Follow workplace procedures when you are required to, but don't let them enslave you. Often there is room for manoeuvre where you can do your own thing as long as you 'pay the rent'.

- Don't devote more time than necessary to the personal goals of others, such as those of your supervisor or employer. Again, 'pay the rent', then act on your own aims and goals. Avoid unnecessary meetings arranged by others. Get people to be clear and specific about why they want the meeting, and be clear as to whether you need to be there. Consider sending a delegate in your place. Ask if issues that involve you could be discussed at a prearranged time so you can deal with them and then leave.[7]

I just can't say 'no'

Does fear of disapproval from others make it hard for you to set limits on how much they use you and your time? Do you believe that putting your priorities first would make you a bad or selfish person, so that fear of guilt leads to passivity?

- Refresh your understanding of the principles of *self-acceptance* (page 58) and *enlightened self-interest* (page 60).

- Remind yourself that *your* goals and time are just as important as anyone else's.

- Use *rational self-analysis* (page 70) to analyse fears about disapproval or guilt.

- Use *exposure* (page 87) — commit yourself to practise saying 'no' (or doing other things you fear might lead to disapproval) at least once a day for a month.

- See Chapter 13 for more help on saying 'no'.

There are too many distractions

Low discomfort tolerance may encourage you to daydream, or get distracted by things that take your eye or attention, in order to put off difficult tasks.

- Enjoy yourself in the present and take regular time out — but resist the temptation to watch just a few more minutes of television or socialise instead of getting started on difficult tasks.

- Put distracting items, such as magazines, light books or personal correspondence, out of sight. Turn off the television and radio (unless you find background music a help).

- Keep Lakien's question (page 255) somewhere in front of you where your eyes tend to alight when you slip into dream mode. (I keep it on top of my computer monitor.)

- Re-train yourself with punishments (such as missing a favourite TV programme) when you have given in to temptation, and with rewards when you go a full day keeping to your schedule.

I can't seem to get things finished

If you find it hard to finish tasks, you may be allowing yourself to get diverted to other things, getting too focussed on the process of doing rather than on the desired outcome, or holding on to a task to wring the last little bit of perfection out of it.

- Keep your goals realistic and settle for excellence rather than perfection. Remember the 80/20 rule. Go for what is good enough.

- Don't schedule more into the day than you can reasonably expect to complete.

- Handle a document once only — action it or file it.

- Break large tasks into smaller bites so you can stay with one task until completed.

- If you have to leave a task unfinished, ensure that you schedule a time to get back and complete it.

- Set deadlines and stick to them.

- Keep Lakien's question (page 255) in front of you.

I find it hard to make decisions on what to do

There are four main reasons why you might have difficulty making decisions: (1) what you *want* to do conflicts with what you think you *should* do; (2) you engage in *black-and-white thinking* — seeking the 'perfect solution' or the 'right' decision; (3) *low discomfort tolerance* makes you avoid the risk involved in committing yourself to a decision; or (4) *lack of self-acceptance* leads you to connect your 'self-worth' with making the 'right' decision.

- Set a time-limit on making your decisions, with a commitment that if you have not decided when the time is up, you will toss a coin and go with whatever the coin shows. Before long you will want to make your own decisions rather than have the coin decide for you.

- Remember that making mistakes does not say anything about you as a *person*.

- Remind yourself that hardly ever is there a 'perfect' solution or only one 'right' course of action, and that it is usually better to risk making a 'wrong' decision than to make no decision at all. (Sometimes, however, it will be appropriate to choose not to decide — just make sure that this is a deliberate choice and not simply avoidance.)

- Seek advice and opinions when you lack some information, but ultimately trust your own judgement.

- Do a *benefits calculation* (page 78) on the advantages and disadvantages of making a decision now or continuing to put it off. Be honest about the real costs and risks of continuing to delay. You can also use this technique to make the decision itself.

- Use *rational self-analysis* (page 70) to identify and combat any demands that conflict with wants.

I keep feeling tired, which slows me down

- Take regular breaks: go for a walk, use a quick relaxation technique, etc — just do something different for a short while.

- Keep a glass of water handy and sip at intervals to keep refreshing yourself.

- To keep the blood circulating, regularly move your body during breaks and while sitting at your workstation.

Nothing seems to work

If you've worked hard at time control but seem to be making no progress, you might be trying to adopt strategies that don't suit your personal style. For example, some people benefit from having a clear desk, whereas others work best with all their files and materials out where they can see them. Are you slavishly trying to follow advice you got from a book, course or colleague, rather than trying different ways of doing things and finding out what works for you?

- To manage time *effectively* you need to know what you want to get out of life. Have you clarified your goals? (See Chapter 12.)

- To manage time *efficiently,* you need to develop strategies suited to your style. An excellent approach to time control that allows for individual differences is described in the book by Sunny Schlenger and Roberta Roesch: *How to be Organized in Spite of Yourself.*[8]

- Finally, be prepared to alter direction if and when you realise you are pursuing the wrong objective or there is a better way to do something. If you accept that changes to plans and scheduling are a normal part of reality, you will be less upset by them.

Michael and Theresa were both able to change their direction: Michael to control his stress, Theresa to achieve what mattered most to her. Both needed to begin by taking the time to step back from what they were doing and reflect on where they were going.

Would it be a good use of your time to pause for a moment and ask: 'Where do I want to go in my life?' 'What is the best way to get there?' and 'Am I going that way?'

16

Money:
who owns you?

Money does make a difference — up to a point. Money provides access to things people want: housing, food, education, material possessions, and so on. You can use money to minimise stress, through better nutrition, medical care, legal advice, recreation and social activities. Just having money available, even if it is not used, may give a subjective feeling of security. Money has the potential to enhance control over one's life.

Unfortunately, many people do not realise this potential. For some, lack of control over their money means they constantly feel pressured by the need for more of it. Others, conversely, become obsessed with accumulating and protecting it. In both cases, instead of controlling their money, the money controls them.

Some people have plenty of money but are still unhappy and stressed, whereas others with little money manage their stress very well. Clearly, then, money *by itself* is not the answer to happiness and control over your life.

The crucial factor is your attitude toward money. Your attitude will influence what you do with your money and how happy you are. Happiness is not determined by the money you have; it is determined by the beliefs you have about your money.

Mark and Sarah, a young couple with two incomes

who wanted to buy their own home and start a family, had developed some unhelpful attitudes that were blocking them from their goals and moving them in the opposite direction to that they wanted, toward increasing indebtedness to others. How they regained control over their money and their future is described in Chapter 19 (on the subject of problem-solving), which can usefully be read in conjunction with this chapter.

Values-based money management

Grady Cash, in his book *Conquer the Seven Deadly Money Mistakes*,[1] invites readers to answer the question: Are you spending in harmony with your deeply felt values? Cash, a financial counsellor, has seen families spending significant sums of money in areas that were never part of their goals or dreams, and this expenditure was destroying their chances of realising those dreams. Over the years as I supervised a community budgeting service, I observed the same pattern: people spending large amounts of money and, far from getting anywhere, slipping deeper into debt and distress.

For your spending to be in line with your values, you need to know what those values are. You need to know what you want out of life. Otherwise your expenditure will be aimless, or simply in reaction to the pressures of the moment.

This is yet another example illustrating the importance of being clear about your goals and values. If you have not yet clarified your goals, see Chapter 12 for help with this. Once you know what your goals are, base your spending decisions on them. Let's say you want to replace your old car. Do you buy a new car or a much cheaper second-hand one? If your most important goal is to achieve status, that might lean you towards the new car. But if your main goal is an overseas trip, you might choose the second-hand model.

You can apply this principle of goal-based spending to all your expenditure — including necessities, such as housing, food, clothing, and so on.

What do we use money for?

Grady Cash points out that money has no value in itself; it is useful only because it can be used to obtain the following four things:

1 *Material items.* These range from survival essentials, such as clothes, housing and food, to less essential items that may add to life, such as a television set, a remodelled kitchen or a nice garden.

2 *Services.* Things such as electricity, medical treatment and car repairs, or being waited on at a restaurant or attending a movie.

3 *Experiences.* Holidays, seeing new places, socialising, meeting new people, learning new things, etc.

4 *Feelings.* People want to have good feelings. Money cannot of course buy feelings directly; but, apart from the necessities of physical survival, people use their money to obtain material items, services and experiences primarily for the feelings that result from having these things. Is it possible that feeling good is the ultimate goal every human being is seeking?

Could you feel just as good as you do now, or even better, by adjusting the ways in which you use money? Which will give you the greatest happiness: spending on expensive restaurants, or eating out more cheaply and using the savings to send a child to university? Upgrading to a more modern computer, or taking music lessons?

Using your money purposefully

Apart from essential spending to meet survival needs, what portion of your spending on material items, services and experiences is for the purpose of having good feelings? Are your current spending patterns actually achieving that purpose, in both the short- and the long-term?

If you want to make the best use of your money, look at your expenditure in each of the following four areas:

1 *Are you paying for material items you could get more cheaply or provide yourself?* Could you heat your house for less by investing in insulation? Could you grow your own vegetables or buy food in bulk and preserve it?

2 *Are you paying more for services than you need to?* Could you learn how to do household repairs or redecorating, get as much enjoyment by eating out at cheaper restaurants, or record television movies instead of hiring videos?

3 *Are you paying more for experiences than you need to?* Buying experiences is often a good use of money. An overseas trip, for example, is like an investment — you may benefit from the memories for many years. But if the point is to see one of the world's great cities, why not stay in a good bed-and-breakfast rather than paying out for staying at an expensive hotel?

4 *Are there some things you could do to achieve greater happiness that involve spending little money, or perhaps none at all?* The ultimate goal is to feel good. Remember that your feelings are not simply the result of what happens in your life — they result from *how you view* what happens.

The real secret to feeling good

If you believe that you 'must' get what you want or that you 'must not' be deprived, then you will be unhappy when you don't have it — and at risk of spending money you can't afford. Let's say, for instance, you believe that you absolutely 'need' the love of your grandchildren. If they appear to be uninterested in you, you may try to buy their love with expensive presents.

Keep in mind that *money alone cannot buy you good feelings.* If the things on which you spend your money give you pleasure, and you can afford the expenditure, then fine. But if you rely on money alone to feel happy, you are at risk, paradoxically, of achieving lower levels of happiness. This is because *to be happy, you need to work on what you think.* Relying on material items, services or experiences will divert your energy from what you really need to do — change how you view the events and circumstances of your life.

Does this open up some ways you could use your finances more productively? Rather than spending money to compensate for feelings of depression, would you be better to learn how to handle negative emotions? Could you stop trying to buy the love of other people, and instead spend more time with them? Rather than spend money to get back at a partner who treats you badly, could you instead learn how to be more assertive with them?

How to achieve more with your money

Operate on a financial plan

The concept of financial planning is straightforward: you record your income and your expenditure, and juggle the two until they balance.

Simply balancing expenditure with income, however, is not the ultimate aim. The financial plan is a tool to help you achieve your goals. Whether the priority is to get out of debt or send a child to university, financial planning is something you do all your life to maintain and improve the quality of your existence.

How do you prepare a financial plan? It is not as difficult as it may sound. Your first step is to make sure, as indicated earlier, that you are clear about your goals. Then you need to collect and record your income and your outgoings.

Next, go through your outgoings. Do they reflect your important goals? Is there some allowance for emergencies and planned maintenance? Have you taken into account such things as medical expenses? Is there any provision for your retirement? If any of the things that are important to you are missing, put them in.

Now add up both your income and your outgoings. It is unlikely they will balance first time. If you are fortunate enough to have more income than outgoings, you will be able to introduce some desired items — perhaps savings for a goal you thought you might have to postpone.

More probably, your outgoings will exceed your income. If so, you have several options. One is to increase your income, if that is possible. Think carefully here. Take care, for example, that you don't cater to a low-priority item — such as paying off an expensive lounge suite — by taking a second job and losing out on the high-priority activity of being with your family.

Usually, you balance a financial plan by reallocating expenditure. Look at the figures. Are you paying more for some things than you need to? Identify the low-priority items and start by cutting those. Are there some items of expenditure that give you a poor happiness return? Cut these too.

When you engage in cost-trimming, make sure your decisions are in line with your identified goals. If you have trouble with this, get some expert assistance (more on this later).

How to make your money go further

There are many ways to stretch the income you already have. Below is a sample culled from my own personal experience and from running a large budgeting service.

- *Plan ahead.* Don't wait until you have to purchase something in a hurry. Anticipate your needs so you can take advantage of specials, or at least shop around.

- *Use credit wisely.* A credit card can be useful, but it can also be a curse. You can take advantage of a bargain or obtain something you need when you don't have the cash immediately to hand; but having the card may lead to unnecessary purchases or high finance costs. The best way to use a credit card is to pay the whole amount owing every month, so as to avoid the high interest charges. If you need temporary credit, pay it off as quickly as you can.

- *Avoid unnecessary financial costs.* Pay bills earlier when there is a discount. Pay credit card accounts in full by the due date, to avoid interest. Don't use a credit card for credit — the interest rate can be crippling. Use other, cheaper sources of finance, such as a bank loan. If using credit has been a problem for you in the past, train yourself to wait and save for items you don't need immediately.

- *Reduce the chance of overspending.* When shopping, don't take more money than you can afford to spend. If using a cheque book or credit card, set a limit and stay within it.

- *Plan your shopping trips.* When you go to the supermarket, take a list of what you intend to buy — and stick to it. Resist additional items that take your fancy. Try to avoid taking children to the supermarket, or make it clear they are not to ask you to buy anything not on the list. Go shopping once a week and get everything you need, to save time and running expenses. Take a calculator and compare prices to see which package sizes are most economical.

- *Save money on holidays and recreation.* Camp rather than use motels. Sleep at home and make day trips to places of interest. Develop recreational activities and fun things to do at home with the family: board games, badminton in the back yard, barbecues (use sausages instead of steak, and pine cones which are free and give more flavour than a fancy, expensive, gas-operated cooker).

- *Eat well without breaking the bank.* Plan your meals a week in advance. Use grocery coupons and specials. Have some meals without meat. Keep fast foods to a minimum — they are expensive and low in nutritional value.

- *Shop around.* Check your insurance coverage to see if you can get a better deal elsewhere, get two or three quotes when your tyres need replacing, and so on.

- *Buy in bulk* — provided the savings are significant and you can use all of what you buy.

- *Grow your own* fruit and vegetables if possible.

- *Learn how to preserve food* and take advantage of good bulk-buys or things you grow yourself (but first check the cost of any preserving materials).

- *Dress well for less.* Buy colour-coordinated clothing you can mix and match. Buy clothes you can wear through all seasons, adding or discarding layers as the seasons change. Buy on sale — but watch out for false economy: don't buy clothes of poor quality or limited versatility. Avoid clothing that requires special and expensive care such as dry-cleaning. Modify an outfit you already own, so that it looks and feels different. Try adding accessories to get a new look. Take care of your clothes so they last and continue to look good.

- *Save money on maintenance.* Keep important mainten-ance up-to-date. Saving on oil changes is a false economy when your car's engine wears out before its time. Delaying house painting may cost you extra to repair weathering damage. Sometimes paying a little more will mean lower maintenance costs and longer life. On other occasions a cheaper item will do the job just as well.

Overcoming the blocks to money control

I never have the money for what I really want

If you don't know what you really want out of life, sensible financial planning will be impossible, and you will be open to manipulation or impulse-buying. Knowing your wants, aims and goals is the starting point to effective financial planning and rational buying decisions.

- Check that your spending benefits both yourself and those important to you. When tempted to buy something not part of your plan, ask yourself these questions: 'Will buying this be in my interests?' 'Will it create problems for other people?' 'What am I prepared to forgo to get it?' 'Will this work out with the important people in my life?'

- Make sure your spending decisions are based on what you really want out of life — not on 'shoulds' or the opinions of others.

It's too uncomfortable to change my spending habits

Low frustration tolerance will lead you to seek short-term gratification rather than long-term gains. It will make it hard to overcome inertia, stop drifting and start planning your life. You may watch television instead of painting the house, or procrastinate over paying your bills.

- Re-study the principle of *tolerance for frustration and discomfort* (page 61). When changing spending habits, resisting the impulse to buy, or facing the dis-comfort of preparing a financial plan, remind yourself that the frustration is unpleasant but not fatal.

- Apply *exposure* (page 87) and *paradoxical behaviour* (page 88). Practise tolerating frustration and dis-comfort. For a while, deliberately postpone any non-essential purchases. Schedule a time to start on that financial plan. Make appointments to see any creditors you can't pay right away.

I don't trust my judgement

If you don't trust your own judgement, you may end up letting others decide what is right for you, or avoid asking for information on products or services through fear that others will think you ignorant.

- Re-study the principle of *self-acceptance and confidence* (page 58). If you accept yourself, you will have less need to buy things just to boost your ego or impress others. You will be less afraid to reveal what you don't know and ask for the information you need to make sensible spending decisions. And you will be able to make mistakes and learn from them without the fear of putting yourself down.

- Trust your own judgement. It's sometimes wise to collect information or seek others' opinions, but in the end, you need to weigh the evidence and decide what is best for you.

I was brought up never to spend money except for absolute necessities

Some people get obsessed with saving money. They travel long distances or search for weeks to find a lower price. They spend hours repairing an item which could be cheaply replaced. They fail to realise that time is valuable too. What are your priority goals? To save money for its own sake — or to put your time into pleasurable and rewarding activities?

- Avoid extravagances when finances are tight, but keep your money-saving activities in proportion. Don't get so obsessed that you forget the point of having money — which is to achieve your goals.

- Recognise the importance of adapting to changing circumstances, and be able to let go of some spending and consuming habits and replace them with others.

I often spend money because I feel bad

People may spend money not because they need what they buy, but for other, usually subconscious purposes: revenge, affection-seeking, to alleviate guilt, lift a depressed mood, boost their own ego or impress others. Unfortunately, the money spent is often wasted. Worse, energy is diverted from learning to deal with emotions in more productive ways.

- Make a habit of planning all purchases in advance,

postponing any inappropriate purchases, and only buying items that are on your list.

- Keep in mind the purpose of forgoing something you want. It is not to make you a person of high moral calibre. The real purpose is more down-to-earth — to obtain greater pleasure later on. Don't forgo that new outfit because it would be 'wrong' — forgo it because you want an overseas trip. This will be more motivating.

- Most importantly, develop your ability to use inexpen-sive techniques such as *rational self-analysis* (page 70) as effective methods to deal with unwanted emotions.

I can't stop compulsive spending

Some people feel compelled to buy things they don't really need without ensuring they have the funds. This can range from compulsively collecting unnecessary items at the expense of more important things, to running up financially crippling credit card accounts. It may start as a way to change bad feelings or compensate for something missing in one's life; as each spending episode temporarily makes the person feel better, an addiction is gradually cemented in place.

- Take control of your own destiny. Dispute any idea that your finances are under the control of magical forces such as 'fate' or 'luck'.

- Don't make yourself a 'victim' by blaming others — your children, partner, employer, bank, the govern-ment — for your difficulties in managing money. Accepting responsibility for your own actions is the first step toward taking control.

- Recognise that the universe is not set up to provide everything you want. If you get rid of any demanding beliefs that you 'should' be able to have such-and-such, or that you absolutely 'need' it, then you will find it easier to keep your spending and your life under control.

- Plan all purchases in advance and, when doing the shopping, stick to the list.

- Practise *postponing gratification* (page 89): allow yourself non-essentials, but delay their purchase.

Further training in financial control

You may find it helpful to increase your knowledge of how to get more from your resources — healthy eating on a budget, do-it-yourself, and so on. You can obtain information from books, adult education classes or your local Citizens' Advice Bureau.

Are you having trouble designing and operating a financial plan? Are you in so much debt you can't see your way out? Most communities have a free budget advisory service which can help you. By the way, avoid the temptation of so-called 'debt-consolidation' firms — they make it sound so easy to get out of debt, but their loan conditions are often crippling.

Some problems will be resistant to self-help. Compulsive spending, gambling, alcohol and drug abuse can be addictions that are hard to break. Don't let these problems continue to wreck your life — get professional help. Try to find a counsellor or therapist who will, rather than dig up your past, help you discover and change whatever keeps you addicted in the present — and show you how to stay free in the future.

Changing the myths about money

There are many beliefs that can keep a person controlled by their money. Here is a representative sample with rational alternatives that will get you started on the road towards being in charge.

Money myths	Rational alternatives
Money is evil.	Money is a means of exchange. I can choose to become obsessed with it — or use it to achieve my goals.
I need money to be happy.	Money is relevant to security and health — but my emotions ultimately result from what I think rather than from what I have.
It's too uncomfortable to stop myself from spending.	It is uncomfortable — but discomfort is a part of real life, and the more I tolerate it the more power and control I gain over myself and my life.
I shouldn't need to plan my spending.	Where is it written that I should be exempt from what most of the human race has to do if they want to get on?
I don't have enough money to operate a financial plan.	I don't have enough money to *not* plan! The less you have, the more you need to plan what you do with it.
If I had more money, I would be more satisfied.	Expectations increase along with income! If I *prefer* to have more but avoid thinking I *must*, I will be satisfied enough to get on with life.

To see how Mark and Sarah, the young couple described at the beginning of this chapter, took control of their money, see Chapter 19.

17

Change:
you can't stop it, but you can steer it

There is nothing new about change. Human beings have always moved through the various stages of the life-cycle, adjusted to bonding with a mate and the arrival of children, become reconciled to the deaths of significant others, and adapted to the ageing process. Such adjustments are still the lot of humans today.

The world, too, has always been changing. For example, I am writing this book on a computer — something I could never have envisaged when I was a child. What is new is the *pace* of change.

Isaac Asimov has said that 'It is change, continuing change, inevitable change, that is the dominant factor in society today.'[1]

Unfortunately, however, as James Baldwin is reported to have said: 'Most of us are about as eager to be changed as we were to be born, and go through our changes in a similar state of shock.'

If both Asimov and Baldwin are correct, then we are faced with two conflicting facts of life. Humans generally dislike change, yet live in world where change is inevitable — and accelerating.

The shock of change

Alvin Toffler graphically described the problems of coping with change in his 1970 book *Future Shock*.[2] He described how people can be psychologically overwhelmed when faced with disaster situations such as major earthquakes, tornados or tidal waves, where homes are wrecked, loved ones killed and lives turned upside down. What is common to such situations is exposure to unfamiliar or unpredictable events and conditions. The senses are bombarded to such an extent that they do not have time to recover from one stimulus before another occurs.

As well as major disasters, everyday events can lead to a feeling of being overwhelmed when a number of changes occur close together. Three years before Toffler's book, Holmes and Rahe published 'The Social Readjustment Rating Scale'[3] which showed how people respond, in terms of their physical and emotional health, to common life events. Some of the items from this scale are reproduced below. The numbers indicate the level of stress associated with a given event, 100 being the highest.

Event	Rating	Event	Rating
Death of a spouse	100	Change in responsibilities at work	29
Marital separation	65	Son or daughter leaving home	29
Marriage	50	Outstanding personal achievement	28
Retirement	45	Trouble with boss or supervisor	23
Pregnancy	40	Change in residence	20
Gaining a new family member	39	Going on holiday	13
Major change in financial state	38	Christmas approaching	12
Changing to a different line of work	36	Minor legal violations	11

You may be surprised to see events listed that most people would not regard as negative. This highlights an important point: even supposedly positive experiences can trigger some level of stress.

Note that the ratings are averages. Your own perception of an event may be different to the rating on the list. Note, too, the scale does not imply that the events and circumstances *themselves* cause stress.

What it shows is that people *perceive* certain events and circumstances in differing ways; and, as we have seen throughout this book, your perception of an event determines how you react to it.

One or a few life events may not lead to significant distress. In fact, some degree of challenge and stimulation is essential to good emotional health. But when a sufficient number of events which are perceived as distressful occur close together in time, a person's coping system may become overloaded — as illustrated with these examples:

- A mid-level manager in a company undergoing restructuring is faced with multiple demands requiring complex decisions. Overload occurs when she has a minor motor vehicle accident shortly after her daughter's wedding.

- A university student is faced with large amounts of information on differing subjects, a number of assignments, and examinations. He experiences overloading when ill-health and problems with flatmates occur close together.

- A homemaker faces demands from children, meal times, the telephone ringing and people calling at the door. The illness of a parent at the same time the family is moving house leads to overload.

Why we need to adapt to change

The world is changing — and will go on changing. A major area of change, as Toffler explains in his book *Powershift*,[4] is the movement from an economy based on capital and manual labour to one based on knowledge and the use of skill. Applying knowledge means less labour, energy, capital, raw materials and time. But this carries a cost. If less physical labour is needed while knowledge and skills grow in importance, then individuals face a need to re-train and adapt to new ways of working.

Another key area of contemporary change is in the way people progress through the life-cycle. As Gail Sheehy points out in *New Passages*,[5] people are taking longer to grow up and longer to die. Consequently, all the stages of adulthood are advancing by up to 10 years. People are having their children later; those in their 40s, 50s and 60s feel five to 10 years younger; and men are increasingly being forced into early retirement. These demographic changes require us to make corresponding changes in our attitudes toward and preparation for the various stages of ageing. Sheehy argues, for instance, that we can now regard age 45 as the beginning of a second adulthood.

If individuals (or societies) try to avoid change, it will still continue around them. They will gradually become further out of touch and isolated from the wider environment. Sooner or later, the environment will have an impact on them in a way that cannot be ignored. Then the adjustment required may be major and disorienting.

At an individual level, you may know people who refuse to adapt, and complain endlessly about how the world has gone, alienating themselves more and more. The same process can happen at a societal or national level. Albania, for instance, was isolated from the rest of the world by its paranoid dictator Enver Hoxhar, who effectively denied his country any chance of participating in the technological advances of the second half of the twentieth century. Albania survived economically by taking handouts, first from Russia and then from China. When these dried up and the Communist regimes in the surrounding countries were overthrown in the 1990s, the Albanian dictatorship eventually collapsed, leaving a poverty-ridden country economically on its knees, with little of the economic infrastructure taken for granted in the rest of Europe.

What this illustrates is that change, uncomfortable though it is, is inevitable — and trying to ignore it provides short-term comfort at the expense of long-term pain.

Change can be managed

Given that change is often stressful, what can you do about it? Fortunately, although it is not possible to prevent change, there are a number of ways in which it can be managed.

Plan for change

You can often ease the impact of change by anticipating and preparing for it. Retirement, for example, is a time when finances are reduced, health problems increase, housing needs change, and there is a substantial increase in spare time. If you save for retirement you can ease the financial pain. Developing a regular fitness and healthy eating routine when you are younger can minimise health problems later. Moving to a smaller, low-maintenance property while you are still mobile will make it easier to establish new relationships. And developing new interests prior to retirement will avoid the boredom that afflicts people for whom physical activities such as work or sport have been the only source of stimulation in their lives.

Space changes

Try to anticipate changes and avoid too many major events occurring close together in time. Some things, such as the death of a loved one, will be unpredictable; but many changes or events can be anticipated and spaced. If a child is leaving home, you might delay changing your job. You could hold off making major financial decisions soon after a bereavement, or postpone upgrading your car when you have just had surgery.

Minimise overstimulation

When you feel overloaded, try to follow familiar, comfortable routines until you get your energy back.

At such times, delegate or postpone decisions. Put off situations which involve meeting new people, and temporarily stick with those you already know and feel comfortable with. Resist unneeded changes in organisations to which you belong (but keep in mind that progressive change and development may be needed to avoid radical change later on).

Make use of support

Support groups can help with negotiating change. They may bring together people going through a similar life transition, such as bereavement, unemployment, separation, new parenthood or retirement. Such groups are not for 'therapy', but for support and mutual help in clarifying goals and sharing strategies for managing the transition. Involvement in such a group is temporary, for as long as it takes the individual to adjust.

Counselling is another form of support. Redundancy, separation and retirement counselling are examples of how people can be helped to deal with change in a structured way.

Maintain personal stability zones

We can cope less stressfully with change by maintaining what Toffler calls 'personal stability zones'. Here are some examples:

- *Retain comfortable and valued elements of your physical environment.* Keep clothes for longer — resist new fashion trends. Keep your car for longer — avoid changing it for minor enhancements. Don't upgrade computer software every time a new version comes out. Keep furniture if it is comfortable and suitable for its purpose; have it reconditioned rather than replaced.

- *Maintain some old friends and acquaintances* with whom you feel comfortable, even as you meet new people. Be open to new experiences, new literature, new music — but have favourite things to fall back on when you need a bit less stimulation.

- *Maintain any daily habits that are usually functional for you*, even when you are out of your normal environment. For example, when travelling, try to go to bed and get up at your usual times, have your daily relaxation period, read before going to bed, or do whatever it is your habit to do.

- *Maintain rituals that provide continuity* in the face of change. As Imber-Black and Roberts explain in their book *Rituals for our Times*,[6] rituals have the capacity to ease difficult life transitions by providing a sense of connection with others and with the past. Many people have become isolated from the rituals they were brought up with, owing to factors such as migration, remarriage or the separation of parents. There may be a need to develop new rituals that are more appropriate and meaningful to the present.

Rituals can apply to daily things such as bedtimes, leaving and returning to the home, leisure activities and how weekends are used; as well as special occasions such as birthdays, relationship anniversaries, reunions, and starting or leaving school. All of these contribute to a sense of continuity, even when the rituals them-selves alter to reflect individual and family changes.

Have more than one source of satisfaction in your life

The more connections you have with the world at large — family, friends, co-workers, church, clubs — the more sources of support you can call on to help manage the stress of change.

These connections, along with your various hobbies and other interests, will also be the sources of satisfaction and enjoyment in your life.

Having multiple sources of satisfaction can be helpful when one area of your life is not going well. You may compensate for stressful changes at work, for example, by continuing to get enjoyment from your children, social activities and other pursuits.

Manage your reactions to change

Finally, and most importantly, keep your emotional reactions in proportion to the changes you are facing. If you have been made redundant, be concerned rather than fearful. When your child is leaving home, feel sad but not depressed. When there are more things to do than time available, be alert but not tense.

Use the strategies of *rational effectiveness training* (Chapter 6) to identify and change the self-defeating thinking that underlies self-defeating emotions and behaviours.

Overcoming the blocks to managing change

I don't know how to deal with the demands of other people

Managing change will be difficult if you find it hard to say 'no' or to ask for what you want. If, for example, the boss wants to schedule a major project when your daughter plans to have her wedding, you will have trouble negotiating if you are afraid to speak up.

- Tell other people when their plans conflict with yours, and negotiate changes to reduce the number of things that happen close together.

- Be prepared to move your own plans when appropriate; when it's not, ask others to move theirs.

- Re-read Chapter 13 for more detailed guidance on how to manage the demands of other people.

Change is too uncomfortable, so I just want to avoid it

Are you prone to viewing some changes as 'awful' or 'unbearable'? Catastrophising about the badness of change will turn concern into anxiety and make you want to avoid or resist it. Established patterns of behaviour provide a sense of comfort and security that change disrupts. You will find it hard to adapt if you have a low tolerance for discomfort.

- Re-study the principles of *tolerance for discomfort* (page 61), *long-range enjoyment* (page 61) and *risk-taking* (page 62).

- Don't resist change or (at the other extreme) be passive towards it: actively embrace it. You will find this easier when you see change as uncomfortable rather than 'unbearable'.

- Change will often be easier to bear if you view it in

a long-term perspective. The *time projection technique* (page 85) can you help with this.

- Many changes will contain an element of risk. Remind yourself that calculated risks are an important part of achieving a stimulating and satisfying life, whereas avoidance of risk is a guarantee of boredom.

- Keep risk-taking in proportion: spacing changes and avoiding unnecessary change are ways of making it a positive rather than a negative experience.

I have a low tolerance for frustration

Low frustration tolerance arises from believing that certain events and circumstances 'should not' or 'must not' occur. Do you hold any beliefs like 'The balance of my life must not be disturbed' or 'I shouldn't have to make adjustments'? Ideas like these will exacerbate anxiety and lead to anger or feelings of hopelessness.

- Re-study the principles of *tolerance for frustration* (page 61), *emotional and behavioural responsibility* (page 63) and *flexibility* (page 64).

- Dispute any idea that you should be exempt from change. View the frustrations involved with change as something to grow with, not a burden to be avoided.

- Take responsibility for how you feel and behave, rather than blame it on other people, the government or fate. This will give you more motivation to influence change, and help you handle your feelings when change does not go the way you want.

- Developing flexibility as a guiding principle in your life will help guard against blind resistance or avoidance. It will help you adapt — to bend with the storm rather than be broken by it.

I don't want change

Non-acceptance of change can show in many ways. Some people, for example, have trouble accepting the ageing process. A woman anxious about physical attractiveness may engage in dangerous dieting as ageing leads to normal weight increase. An older man over-concerned with physical performance may run the risk of injuries by continuing to play contact sports.

- Re-study the principles of *self-acceptance* (page 58) and *acceptance of reality* (page 65).

- Work on accepting yourself irrespective of your changing appearance or abilities. Enjoy being an older person instead of denying the reality of passing youth. Focus on maximising the quality of your life now, rather than trying to re-live the past.

- When change is in the air, don't deny or avoid it — get involved. Join the committee set up to implement change at your workplace. Get to know the local member of parliament and express your views. Write to newspapers. Start a neighbourhood action group. Use your energy not to avoid change, but rather to influence it in a productive direction. Sometimes it will be in your interests to *initiate* change rather than just respond to it. If you are bored with your job, don't complain — ask for changes, or consider a new job or even a change of career. If there are inefficiencies at work, don't wait for others to impose change — initiate it yourself.

- Finally, some changes will be negative experiences for you, and out of your control. But you still have a choice about how you react to them. You can rail against fate and spend the rest of your life consumed with bitterness. Or you can choose to grieve for your loss, pick yourself up, and get on with life. Don't resist change — or ignore it.

Changing your beliefs about change

How you manage the changes in your life will depend, mainly, on what you tell yourself about it. Here are some of the most common self-defeating beliefs about change, along with rational alternatives.

Change myths	Rational alternatives
The world is getting worse.	Some things are getting worse, some things are getting better.
I can't stand to have my life disrupted.	I dislike disruption, but obviously I can stand it — it has happened many times and I am still alive to tell the tale!
Life should be predictable and certain.	Life has never been predictable and certain — where is it written that it should be so now?
It would be selfish to ask others to change their plans when they conflict with mine.	It is enlightened to take into account the wishes of others; self-interested (rather than 'selfish') to do the same with mine.
It is easier to avoid change and its discomfort and pain.	It is (sometimes) easier in the short-term to avoid change. But this makes it harder later on.
I can't help feeling bad in response to the changes in my life.	How I feel in response to change depends on what I tell myself about it. And I can have control over my beliefs.
What will happen will happen, so you can't influence change.	If I believe this, I will most likely end up proving my own prophecy!
To be unchanging shows stability and strength.	Resisting change demonstrates anxiety and rigidity. Working with and influencing change shows courage and flexibility.

As Aldous Huxley wrote in his *Collected Essays,* 'Enlightenment is not for the quietists and puritans who, in their different ways, deny the world, but for those who have learned to accept and transfigure it.'[7]

18

Balance:
is there enough in your life?

The human body requires constant change in order to function. Consider your sense of smell. When you scent a rose, you are struck by the lovely perfume. After a while, however, the intensity diminishes as your sense of smell adjusts. If you go to a different type of rose, you can smell once again — because your nose finds the scent new and novel.

The brain works on the same principle: it constantly needs re-stimulating. Notice how reading a book at first seems absorbing, but then your concentration begins to dull. However, when you put the book down and do something else for a while, you come back to it fresh.

Lack of variety and stimulation leads to boredom. This state of mental weariness and discontent is itself stressful. Boredom may lead to depression, or to high levels of frustration which can trigger aggression. There is a paradox here: we usually think that having too many things going on increases the risk of losing control over our lives, but not having enough variety can lead to the same end.

A degree of challenge and stimulation is important to your mental health. When stress rises too high, performance begins to decline. Both of these are true. You need challenge — and the occasional break from challenge.

Michael, whom we met earlier in the book, was getting plenty of challenge but had lost the balance in his life. Since his promotion to management, he was spending increasing time at work trying to cope with a role for which he was ill-prepared. He had stopped going to the gym, arrived home after his children had gone to bed, and worked most weekends. It was only after he went to his doctor with a variety of physical symptoms that were diagnosed as stress-related, and his wife Amanda warned him that their marriage was at risk, that Michael realised how out-of-balance his life had become.

How you can create stimulation and variety

Introduce variety into your workday

'Work' is what you do to earn a living or maintain yourself and your dependants. It may involve housework, a business you operate from home, or a job in an office or factory.

Introducing variety into your workday in the form of *pauses* — breaks at regular intervals through the day — can improve your concentration and functioning. The extent to which you can do this will depend on how much control you have over your workday. This was an important message for Michael. Once he realised that time away from work would increase his efficiency and help him get more done, not less, it was easier for him to commit to changing his lifestyle.

Where control is low, try to get away from your work area whenever you have a scheduled break. Do something entirely different. Have a brief nap, go for a short walk, get some refreshments, read a book, write a letter, socialise with a colleague, listen to music, use a relaxation technique. Taking time out every few hours will refresh you and keep you alert — and help you maintain peak efficiency.

Where you have greater freedom to plan your day, use

it to alternate tasks that take time. 'A change is as good as a rest' may be a rather shop-worn phrase, but it is still true. Take regular breaks to talk to colleagues, get a drink of water, or even just walk to the filing room to get away from your desk.

If you work at home, plan your day so you are not constantly doing the same thing. Take regular breaks from routine tasks such as cleaning and cooking, or home maintenance activities such as painting or redecorating (unless you find them absorbing).

Have interests outside of your work

Have some pursuits that regularly take your mind in a different direction to work. This will help you return to your labour refreshed and with increased efficiency. Common pursuits include such things as:

- sport (organising, playing, coaching, supporting)
- other outdoor activities (walks, beach, picnics, etc)
- an absorbing hobby
- do-it-yourself projects
- organising events (family reunion, concert, dance, play, or sporting event)
- researching (a topic of interest, family history, etc)
- expanding your areas of interest and learning (learning a new musical instrument, meeting new people, and so on)
- an absorbing commitment (volunteer work, committee membership, political activity, writing a book)
- reading, movies, visiting places of interest
- socialising with family or friends
- special treats (like taking a long bath, getting out the photo albums, and so on).

Take planned holidays

If you wait until you have the time, holidays may never happen. If you don't plan ahead, you may waste precious time. Don't wait for holidays to happen — organise them.

Holidays don't have to be spent away from home. You could plan an interesting do-it-yourself project, arrange picnics or visits to a museum or art gallery, call on friends you don't normally get to see, or pursue any number of special activities.

Sometimes you might want to get away from it all. Planning is especially important when bookings need to be made or arrangements need to be set in place to care for your house or pets (or children). Going away can range from a world trip to an inexpensive camping holiday.

Whatever you do, the trick to taking time off is planning. Don't just drift along. Organise your time off work and plan what you are going to do. Then do it.

Finding new things to do

From time to time, vary the things you do and add new pursuits, including items you would not previously have thought of. There are many places to look for ideas.

Your local public relations centre may have a list of events for the next year. Watch notice-boards in supermarkets, church halls, museums and other public places. Many organisations place advertising in public libraries.

Seek out local community groups which offer activities ranging from such things as craft-work, sports and eating out in small groups, through to voluntary helping, such as budget advising or telephone counselling. Free local newspapers are often a rich source of advertisements for community groups and their activities.

If you have lived in the same place for some time, you may have come to take it for granted and could be surprised to discover just what is happening all around you.

Getting into action

If you are not used to taking time out, it may be especially important to plan recreation rather than wait until you 'have time'. Planning ahead can help you combat the tendency of most human beings towards inertia, which we will discuss shortly.

Recreation activities sheet

An activity planner like the one below will help get you started. Develop some kind of recreational activity for each day of the next week, and record in each square what you plan to do for that day. Some days you will have time for only a short activity; on other days you will be able to set aside time for a longer one. It is fine to repeat an activity, so long as it is not so repetitive that it becomes boring. Here is an example (from Michael's plan):

Saturday	Sunday	Monday	Tuesday	→ etc
Clean car.	AM: Church.	Gym.	Brendan's school concert.	
Sort fishing gear.	PM: Fishing with Brendan.	Watch TV movie.		
Mow lawns.	Watch TV documentary.			
PM: Family to movies.				

At the end of each week, review what you have done. Tick the items you carried out, and put a cross by the ones you missed. Analyse why you missed these activities. There may be a valid reason —for example, there was an unexpected opportunity to substitute a better activity. But watch for invalid reasons, such as 'I didn't have time' (especially when the reason appears more than once). Plan how you can get around any blocks. Keep using the chart until you find that you are routinely making time for recreation.

Michael found the activities sheet useful. He had become so locked in to his work that he found it hard to think of things to do outside of the workplace. Planning his non-work activities at the beginning of each week provided some structure that helped him break the old pattern. He also involved Amanda in the planning process. This meant she could suggest activities (especially helpful in the early stages when Michael found it hard to think creatively), and it also helped him re-engage with his wife and family. In addition, because she was aware of Michael's plan for each week, Amanda was able to remind him to stick with it when he began to worry about his work again.

Overcoming the blocks to an energising life

Given that human beings are usually motivated to seek pleasure and avoid pain, it may seem strange that we would need to talk about blocks to self-enjoyment. The reality is that many people have self-defeating attitudes and behaviours that get in the way.

I feel guilty when I do things just for enjoyment

If you feel guilty about pleasure, you will keep putting work or other people ahead of yourself. Beliefs such as the following will often underlie guilt: 'It's wrong to put pleasure before work', 'You can't relax until all the work is up-to-date' (I would never relax if I believed this!), 'You should always put other people first' or 'I don't deserve to enjoy myself.'

- Apply the principle of *self-acceptance* (page 58). Get rid of the idea that you have to 'deserve' pleasure or 'earn' it. Seek activities that are enjoyable in themselves, not because they prop up your self-image.

- Watch for any over-competitiveness, fear of failure, or anxiety about your reputation that creeps into your recreational pursuits.

- If you accept yourself, you will be able to feel comfortable with your own company, and thus enjoy a greater range of recreational options.

- Practise *enlightened self-interest* (page 60). For variety and stimulation to do you much good, it needs to be the kind you want — not what suits someone else. There are times when compromise is called for, such as going on a picnic with the family when you would rather surf the Internet, but make sure you are not constantly fitting in with others' plans to the exclusion of your own. Remember, balance is the aim.

I don't have time for pleasure

Most of us, if we are going to find time for anything, need to *make* that time. If you wait until you 'have time' for recreation, it will hardly ever happen. Are you constantly responding to external demands rather than taking control of your time?

- Know what you like and know what you want to get out of life. Then you will put your time and energy into activities that will bring you the most rewards.

- Don't wait until you have time — *make* time to do the things you really enjoy. How you spend your time is a matter of how you choose to set your priorities. What you think you 'have' to do is, in reality, a choice. You can choose to make enjoyable activities a high priority. See Chapter 15 if you need some help with controlling time.

- Accept that you can't do everything. If you are like me, your work will never be 'up-to-date' (whatever that means!). Accept that reality, and get on with putting more variety and stimulation into your life.

I can try only things where success is guaranteed

Do you distrust your intelligence or abilities? If so, you will restrict the range of activities open to you. A strong fear of failing will also make you less likely to try new things. Or it could lead you to become over-competitive, which will take much of the enjoyment and relaxation out of your recreation. When we say we are afraid of failing, what we really mean is that we fear disapproval from others and our own self-downing. Sitting beneath this is lack of self-acceptance.

- Review the principle of *self-acceptance* (page 58). Remember that you don't become a different person when others disapprove of you, and that failing does not make you (as a person) a 'failure'.

- *Self-knowledge* (page 58) is also important. Know what you are capable of and what your limits are. Then you will make sensible choices on recreational activities without unnecessarily restricting your options. Do you have a disability? Changing attitudes toward disability, and advances in equipment such as lighter and stronger wheelchairs, open up a widening range of activities and lead to increases in confidence for people with disabilities. Maximise your options, but don't set yourself up for disillusionment with unreasonable expectations.

- Re-study the principle of *risk-taking* (page 62). There

are risks involved in stepping out and trying new things. But you guarantee lower satisfaction if you play it safe and only ever pursue what you already know. Risk-taking is part of a stimulating and variety-full life. Don't just think about doing something different. Try it out. Some things will work for you, some will not; but there is no way of knowing without trying them.

I can't tolerate being alone

If you have an excessive fear of loneliness, you may cut yourself off from many enjoyable activities that involve being alone. Spending time with other people is important to most human beings; but spending some time alone will provide variety and refreshment in your life (making your socialising, when you engage in it, even more enjoyable). See page 246 for suggestions on overcoming loneliness.

I tend to get carried away and overdo things

If you take an enjoyable activity and become obsessed with it, then it will lose its pleasure and become a new source of stress. Do you exercise compulsively, spend all night on the Internet, or find you can't put down a book or magazine until you have read it right through?

- Re-study the principle of *moderation* (page 62). Exercise is good for you, in moderation. Enjoy watching television, but don't become a couch potato. Get inspiration from involvement in a political or community action group, but remain able to see other points of view.

- Practise *flexibility* (page 64). Don't get in a rut. Avoid doing things the same old way all the time. Go to work by a different route some days. Skip the cafeteria now and again; bring your lunch from home and eat it under the trees. Go camping in a different place next holidays. Be able to move from one activity to another in order to maintain your freshness, enjoyment and efficiency.

I just can't break out of my inertia

It is often easier to think about doing something than to do it — even when the activity is potentially enjoyable. Human beings seem to have a natural tendency towards inertia. Underlying this, mostly, is low discomfort tolerance.

- Review the principle of *tolerance for frustration and discomfort* (page 61). Remind yourself that while overcoming inertia is uncomfortable, it is not fatal — and will get easier the more you do it.

- Aim for *long-range enjoyment* (page 61). Acknowledge the reality that highly satisfying pursuits — such as learning a musical instrument, writing a book, or building a house — take time to develop and bear fruit, but will increase your long-term life-enjoyment.

- Re-study the principle of *commitment* (page 63). People benefit from having a variety of activities. With some, such as attending a movie, you will have only a superficial commitment. But greater satisfaction will come from absorbing yourself in one or a few undertakings on a long-term basis.

- Practise *behavioural responsibility* (page 63). Blaming your boss or partner because you don't seem to have time for yourself is a sure way to remain stuck. Take responsibility for your own action or lack of it. When you see that making your life more interesting is in your own hands, you will have taken the first step toward doing something about it.

Boredom or stimulation?

Unbalanced beliefs	Rational alternatives
It is self-indulgent and weak to seek pleasure when there is work to be done.	Variety and stimulation are important to physical and mental health — and they help me work smarter rather than harder.
You should always get your work up-to-date before you play.	Sometimes it is appropriate to discipline myself to complete a task before playing. But my work can never be 'up-to-date'. And taking breaks makes me more efficient in the long run.
It is easier to just drift along with whatever happens rather than try to change anything.	It is only easier in the short-term. Inertia leads to boredom and depression. Facing the immediate discomfort of getting moving will make life better in the long-term.
I can't take time for myself because other people make it impossible.	Other people may make things difficult, but ultimately I choose whether I fit in with them — or seek what I want.
I don't have the time to take time out.	How I allocate my time is, ultimately, a matter of choice.

Problems:

when they come, know what to do

We are constantly solving problems. Much of the time we do this unawares; at other times we consciously grapple with a dilemma. Picking an ice-cream flavour, deciding what to have for dinner, balancing the budget, choosing a career, dealing with a difficult child, or finding a retirement home are all examples of problem-solving.

The central theme of this book is that distress results from how we view things rather than from problematical events and circumstances themselves. Where, then, does problem-solving fit? It is true that changing beliefs is the most dependable route to control over our lives — but if we can also change the activating events themselves, and get more of what we want (and less of what we don't), so much the better.

The problem-solving process

Mark and Sarah were a young couple with two incomes who wanted to buy their own home and start a family. Unfortunately, these goals seemed to be eluding them because they were not saving any money; in fact, they were moving increasingly into debt.

What do you do when a problem is difficult to solve and requires a calculated search for solutions? The answer is to consciously use a structured approach. This involves going through a series of steps: defining the problem, getting information, developing courses of action, putting them into practice, and evaluating the results. This is what Mark and Sarah needed to do. They had been saying: 'We must save more', 'We need to spend less' or 'Maybe we should get second jobs', but without seriously considering any options or actually doing anything.

In my earlier book, *Choose to be Happy*,[1] I described a structured problem-solving process in detail. What follows is a summarised version of that process. It is one you can use when you have problems that require major decisions, or when there is no obvious course of action.

Some problems can be dealt with quickly, in which case you don't have to go through all the stages. Other issues, especially those that involve major changes in your life, could warrant spreading the process over days or even weeks. Mark and Sarah's problem required more attention than they were giving it.

Step 1. Stop!

When faced with a difficult problem, don't panic and do the first thing that comes to mind — or, at the other extreme, procrastinate to avoid the discomfort involved. If your emotions are running high, sort out your mind before trying to sort out the problem. Completing a *rational self-analysis* (page 70) is a good way to achieve this. If you feel uncomfortable whenever you think about the problem, and put it from your mind to avoid the discomfort, uncover and deal with the low discomfort-intolerance beliefs involved (see page 38).

Step 2. Spell out the problem

State the problem in concrete terms. Be specific: 'Our average weekly expenditure is $300 more than our income' is better than 'We can't make ends meet.' Also, break the problem down into its various parts. This will help you see it more clearly and be able to work on it in small chunks. Be very clear as to exactly what it is you see as problematical.

Mark and Sarah analysed their problem as consisting of four main components: (1) 'Although we both have good incomes we don't seem to know where the money is going'; (2) 'We currently owe a lot of money to a variety of creditors'; (3) 'Interest and credit charges add greatly to our costs'; and (4) 'We are not saving anything.'

Step 3. Collect information

To develop effective solutions, you require information. Here is a process to help with collecting relevant information:

1 *Identify what information you need.* After you have defined the problem, ask this question: 'What do I need to know to reach a solution?'

2 *Identify possible sources of information*: your own past experience, other people, community education classes, organisations, books, magazines, audio- or video-tapes, the Internet, etc.

3 *Access the sources* you have identified.

4 *Extract the information.* Be selective: try to record only relevant information; and summarise it so you are not overwhelmed by facts.

5 *Synthesise the information.* Put together the separate pieces of information you have obtained to form a new combination that addresses the problem.

Mark and Sarah followed this sequence:

1 They decided that some way of keeping track of their finances was required, along with ways to reduce current debt and avoid incurring further debts.

2 They then talked to some friends who had recently moved into their own home, and found a money management site on the Internet.

3 They discovered that their friends had, soon after their marriage, set up a financial plan which helped them control their spending and save. From the Internet they obtained instructions on how to set up such a plan. They also came across information on the real cost of credit, which they had never previously stopped to consider.

4 Putting all this information together suggested some options that were available and assisted them to set some goals.

Step 4. Set goals

Set a direction in which to go by turning the problems into goals. State them as specifically as possible, so that you can know when they have been achieved. 'Be able to keep our spending within our income and save $2,000 per year' is a goal that can be objectively measured. Mark and Sarah set the following goals:

- Set up and operate a financial plan.

- Pay off all our current debts within 12 months, then begin saving.

- Have $30,000 for a house deposit saved within three years.

Don't settle on your final goals until you have considered all the things you might wish for — even the fanciful ones.

'I wish our creditors would all disappear' may be unlikely, but it might trigger some creative thinking that could lead to 'Maybe we could set up a creditors' pool.'[2]

Step 5. Develop alternative solutions (strategies)

Develop a range of possible strategies to achieve the goals you have set. Use the *brainstorming* procedure: write down every potential solution you can think of, no matter how way-out they seem. The idea is to generate the largest number of options you can. Don't criticise any or attempt to analyse how workable they are. At this stage, go for quantity rather than quality. 'Go busking for money' deserves a place alongside 'Draw up a financial plan.' Even apparently way-out ideas may serve to trigger other, more realistic ones. Then decide which strategies to pursue. Carefully examine all the options you have written down, asking three key questions about each:

1 What are the likely *consequences* — both negative and positive, for myself and significant others, both long- and short-term?

2 How does it fit with my *personal value system*?

3 How *useful* would it be in helping me achieve the goal I have set? This is where you decide that busking is out because you can't sing very well!

A single strategy might be enough to achieve a goal, or you might need to follow several courses of action before you get there. Sometimes there will not be any solution which is desirable — the best you can do is decide which would be the least unsatisfactory option.

Mark and Sarah considered a number of strategies relating to all three of their goals. The following strategies relate to goal 1 — Pay off all our current debts within 12 months:

- Contact that debt consolidation company we saw advertised on TV, then we would only have one creditor to pay.

- Go to the local budgeting service and have them run a creditors' pool for us.

- Run a creditors' pool ourselves.

- Sell one of our vehicles (the sports utility vehicle we never take off-road that we purchased on credit with no deposit, and which uses twice as much gas as our little hatchback).

- Cut up all our credit cards so we don't incur any more costs than what we have already.

They decided against option 1, attractive though it seemed at first, after reading that many 'debt consolidation' firms are loan sharks who charge inflated fees and interest rates. They elected to set up a creditors' pool themselves, falling back on the budgeting service if unsuccessful. They were not keen to sell the sports utility vehicle, partly because of the status they perceived it gave them, but also because the value had dropped since fuel prices had risen. However, they decided to go ahead and sell it, as that would get rid of their major debt and save on running costs. They were also unhappy about giving up their credit cards, but research on the Internet had shown them the high interest charge incurred by that form of credit, so they got the scissors out.

Step 6. Identify any blocks to your strategies
Are there any things which might get in the way of the strategies you have chosen? Identify them now, and look for ways to get around them.

Mark and Sarah discovered that the loan contract for the

sports utility vehicle had a clause imposing a punitively high penalty for early repayment. However, the free legal advice service at their local Citizens' Advice Bureau helped them escape the unreasonable clause. The only block to cutting up their credit cards was their own discomfort about having to live within their means, which they dealt with by identifying and changing the 'catastrophic' thinking involved.

Step 7. Develop tasks

By now, you will have one or more strategies aimed at achieving your general goal. You could describe these strategies as *sub-goals*. Now it is time to generate some tasks: specific ways of achieving your strategies or sub-goals. Tasks are what you actually *do*.

For the strategy 'Run a creditors' pool ourselves', Mark and Sarah developed the following tasks:

- List our remaining debts and how much we need to pay each month.

- Complete our financial plan (another goal which had its own set of tasks).

- Draw up a sheet of paper on which to record all payments and amounts still owing.

- Open a special bank account to operate the pool from.

Once again, use the brainstorming method described in step 5, go for the maximum quantity of ideas. Then select the tasks to put into action. Guide your selection with similar questions as for step 4. What are the likely *consequences* of each one? How does it *fit* with my personal value system? Will it be *useful* in achieving the strategy concerned? Also ask: Will this tactic get around the potential blocks I have identified?

Step 8. Act on your tasks

Now carry out the tasks you have chosen.

Step 9. Evaluate the results

If you do not get the results you want, don't give up. Just go back to an earlier stage of the process and start again from that point.

Mark and Sarah found that after recording the monthly amount they required to pay all their creditors, the outgoings on their financial plan exceeded their income. They went back to step 5 and developed an additional strategy: to sell a set of golf clubs Mark had inherited from his grandfather, using the money to pay off a hire-purchase agreement that had high monthly payments. This was followed by step 6 where Mark acknowledged his sense of loss and worked through it by thinking about the long-term gains of having a home of his own and the family he and Sarah both wanted.

How to make decisions

As you will have seen from the experience of Mark and Sarah, an important part of problem-solving is deciding between alternatives. What follows is a technique that puts a structure on what might otherwise seem to be a daunting process. It is the *benefits calculation* referred to earlier in this book (page 78), applied to decision-making.

Draw up a chart like the one on the next page. You can have addit-ional columns for further options if neces-sary. Under each option, list its advantages and disadvantages. Give each of these a weighting according to how important it is to you: 1 for the least important, 10 for the most. Calculate a total for each option by adding up the 'advantages' ratings and subtracting the 'disadvantages' ratings.

	OPTION 1: Go bankrupt	Weight	OPTION 2: Get budgeting help	Weight
Advantages	Wipe out all our debts, make a fresh start.	9	Repay all our debts, even though slowly.	9
	No more pressure from creditors.	8	Learn how to manage money and stay out of debt.	10
		+17		+19
Disadvantages	We would not be able to leave the country.	2	It would take a long time to repay our debts.	7
	We would be barred from starting another business.	7	We would have to expose our incompetence with money to other people.	6
	Creditors would never get paid, this would be hard for some of them.	8		
	We would not learn anything about handling money.	9		
		−26		−13
	Total	−9	Total	+6

Note that advantages and disadvantages include both consequences that are *practical* (for example, 'Would save money') and *emotional* (for example, 'Would feel resentful').

Totalling each column of ratings and comparing the results will help you decide which option to take; although sometimes it is a good idea to look beyond the numbers and see how you feel about each option at a 'gut level'. If your intuition tells you something different to what the numbers say, ask yourself if you have been entirely honest with all your ratings.

When there is more than one problem

It is usually best to deal with problems in order of needs first, then desires. Satisfaction of a higher-level *desire* is unlikely when lower-level *needs* are unmet. Social desires are not likely to be an issue when you are lacking food. Developing a talent will usually take second place to finding somewhere to live.

Trying to solve more than one problem at a time may leave you feeling overwhelmed. If you pick off your problems one by one, you will have a much better chance of dealing with them effectively. Separate and prioritise them so the most important get dealt with first. If you worry about problems being forgotten, make a record of those you are putting on hold.

Overcoming the blocks to solving problems

Below is a list of some of the more common obstacles that may get in the way of problem-solving. Fortunately, all can be overcome.

My life is not under my direction

If you believe your life is under the control of external forces, you may see little point in trying to change anything.

- Give up the magical thinking that leads you to put your head in the sand and rely on mystical forces such as 'fate' to direct your life. See *self-direction* (page 63).

- Review the principle of *emotional and behavioural responsibility* (page 63). No matter what the cause of a problem, keep in mind that you are responsible for what you do about it. This will help you move from blaming to solving. Also, by taking responsibility for how you feel, you can avoid upsetting yourself more than you need to.

- Don't see yourself as a 'victim'. Rather than sit around

blaming or waiting to be rescued, start looking at possible solutions. Use others for advice and support, but in the end make your own decisions on what is to be done. Except when there is good reason to have someone else do it, action those decisions yourself.

I don't seem to know what's important to me

To make decisions and develop solutions that will be right for you, they need to be in line with your values. Knowing your goals and values will help you make decisions you can live with. See Chapter 12 if you need help with this.

What I want conflicts with what I should do

You will have trouble making decisions when there is a conflict between what you *want* to do and what you think you *should* do. To break through the 'shoulds', study the principle of *enlightened self-interest* again (page 60). This will help you judge potential solutions according to how they facilitate your interests, while taking into account how they affect other people.

I need to be sure I get the 'right' solution

Black-and-white thinking could lead you to believe that solutions and decisions are either 'completely right' or 'completely wrong', and that you must always find the 'right' one. However, because there is no such thing as a perfect solution, your internal demand for one could paralyse you from doing anything at all.

- Start by reviewing the principle of *flexibility* (page 64). Remind yourself that there are no black or white answers.

- Judge potential solutions on their level of usefulness, not on their 'rightness'.

- Be open to a range of options. In a rapidly changing world, it is often necessary to look beyond old solutions.

If I make the wrong decision, I will feel bad about myself

If you connect your 'self-worth' with doing things 'right' and never making mistakes, you will be tempted to avoid action because your self-image could be on the line. If you fear disapproval from other people of what you do, you will be even less likely to get into action. And if you regard yourself as less important than others, you are likely to keep putting their interests ahead of your own.

- Review the principle of *self-acceptance* (page 58): give away the idea that you have to be a 'worthwhile' human being, and that being worthwhile depends on your performance and getting approval from others.

- Re-study the principle of *enlightened self-interest* (page 60), then ask yourself how it is that the interests of others are more important than your own.

I can't trust my own judgement

If you don't trust your own opinions, you are likely to become paralysed when trying to decide what to do, or leave it to others to decide for you.

- Review the principles of *confidence* (page 58) and *risk-taking* (page 62).

- Seek opinions from other people, but in the end make up your own mind about what is best for you.

- Acknowledge that nothing is guaranteed, and that taking calculated risks is essential to getting anywhere.

- Use a *benefits calculation* (page 319) to check out the risks and benefits of particular options.

It's easier to just put off doing anything

Sometimes the only viable solution may be uncomfortable to implement. Also, there are risks involved in committing yourself to a course of action and carrying it out: you might start something you can't finish, or things could turn out badly. Accordingly, you may choose the 'safe' path of avoiding the discomfort by doing nothing.

To weigh one thing against another creates internal conflict. Further, to decide on one option means letting go of the others. Low frustration tolerance may keep you holding on to all the options — thus choosing none.

- Re-study the principle of *tolerance for frustration and discomfort* (page 61). Challenge the idea you should be able to lead a life free of problems and should not have to make difficult decisions or carry out uncomfortable actions. When you expect frustration and discomfort, paradoxically they become easier to handle.

- Review the principle of *long-range enjoyment* (page 61). Ensure that problem-solving takes account of your long-term interests rather than simply providing quick relief. With each option, consider whether it will make things better or worse in the long run.

- Accept that making decisions and acting on them usually involves some risk. Ask yourself: 'Is the risk of doing the wrong thing as harmful to my interests as doing nothing?' (See *risk-taking* on page 62.)

- There will always be some problems that cannot be resolved. But there is still an ultimate solution. As the principle of *acceptance of reality* (page 65) shows, if you change what you can and accept what you can't, you will avoid paralysing yourself with bitterness or hopelessness.

Mark and Sarah stopped putting off action on their problem. They accepted the reality that to achieve the goals that mattered most to them, they would have to let some other things go. Uncomfortable though that was at the time, they now have no regrets about trading off short-term pain for long-term gain. Following a structured and logical series of steps helped them take back control over their future.

Are you sitting on one or more problems that you can't see a way through? The answer is to take it step-by-step. Why not take the first step to control right now?

Your job:

personal control in the workplace

Work is an area of life that for many people seems out of their control. People who work for somebody else will have issues that differ from those who work for themselves, but both are liable to feel that their work is taking them over.[1] Michael (introduced in Chapter 9) provides a vivid illustration of loss of control in the workplace. This chapter will show you how to maximise your personal control either as an employee or as the boss, whether you work in a factory, an office, a hospital or a building site. Although it will emphasise the organisational setting, most of the material presented is just as relevant to people who work on their own.

The chapter will also extend the issue of control beyond simply coping. The principles in this book, as well as helping at a personal level, can be used to enhance work performance and increase organisational effectiveness. Applying control to the workplace could easily take up a whole book, but this chapter will summarise some key aspects.

Stress at work

Just about every strategy for personal and life management presented throughout this book applies to the workplace as much as to any other setting. There is, however, a particular type of stress which is a risk factor at work. Known as 'burnout', it is described in detail in an earlier chapter (see page 22). Burnout is characterised by three main stages, typically beginning with a person becoming over-involved with their work and eventually progressing, if untreated, to an opposite state where they may completely reject their occupation.

Recognising the early signs of burnout will enable corrective action. Prevention is even better than cure: you can avoid even the early stages of burnout by practising the personal control strategies described throughout this book.

Getting support at work

A key way to reduce stress at work is to maintain good relationships with others in the workplace. This allows you to get help with problem-solving, avoid feelings of alienation, and operate better as part of a team. Unfortunately, in many work settings, a range of factors can create isolation between workers:

- *Time.* If the workplace is busy, maintaining relationships may seem to be of low priority. People moving up the promotional ladder are especially prone to becoming 'too busy' to take time out to give and receive support.

- *Differences in status and power.* If you are in authority over someone, then you have more power than that person. Subordinates are only too aware that you can recommend for or against their promotion, enhance or reduce their work satisfaction, and, ultimately, play a part in terminating their employment. This power differential makes it hard (and, mostly, undesirable) for managers to seek personal support from their subordinates.

- *Few peers available.* If you are in an executive position, there may be few people at your level easily available to you. This becomes progressively worse as you move further up the ladder. Any competition among peers will make mutual support even more unlikely.

- *The assumption that support should 'just happen'.* People in the workplace often assume that integration into a group, and the giving and taking of support, are things that naturally happen. Consequently, they may do little to see that a new person is included, or take notice when a colleague begins to become isolated.

Make time

It is incorrect to say that we do not have time. We always have time — 24 hours a day of it, 7 days a week, 52 weeks a year. We use that time for whatever we regard as important.

You can choose to see support in the workplace as a priority, and allocate time to it. In fact, time spent on support is time well spent. Reducing stress increases efficiency and effectiveness.

Allow time for informal visiting and chatting with peers and subordinates. Linger behind after a meeting with a colleague. Talk to co-workers during your breaks and take other opportunities to socialise with them.

If you have difficulties with time control, you will find some help with this in Chapter 15.

Look for support in many places

As well as informal contacts, consider having formal meetings with co-workers about your own or shared concerns. Arrange a regular meeting with a supervisor or mentor at which you can deal with issues on a continuing basis. Take opportunities to meet with people in your field from other workplaces, at conferences, seminars, workshops or interest-group meetings.

Return the favour

You can increase the likelihood of support from others if you offer them support. The principle of *enlightened self-interest* (page 60) is just as relevant to the workplace as it is to your personal life.

Maintain appropriate boundaries

If you are a manager or supervisor, communication with subordinates can help ease any sense of isolation, but it is important to maintain *some* boundaries. It may be appropriate to problem-solve with subordinates on matters to do with the workplace, but not to seek their help with your own emotional issues. Save these for your peers, partner or non-work friends.

Be wary of developing an intimate relationship at work. Between peers, there may be some advantages: co-workers are easy to meet, you can learn about them before committing yourself, and they are likely to be similar in socioeconomic status, education and income level. But there are some dangers:[2]

- An attempt to start a romance may be construed as sexual harassment, even if one party thought they were receiving encouragement from the other. Charges of sexual harassment are more likely when there is inequality in status and power between the people concerned.[3]

- A proportion of workplace romances are extramarital affairs, which creates stress both in and out of the workplace.

- A romantic connection between manager and subordinate can be dangerous to both parties. Because of the power differential, it will not be an equal relationship. Co-workers may become jealous. If the relationship ends, one of the parties may have to leave the workplace.

If a supportive relationship at work develops into something more, stand back and ask: Is this in my interests, or would I better to re-establish the boundary?

Cultivate feedback

An important aspect of support at work is feedback on one's personal performance. Unfortunately, it is not easy to get honest feedback, usually because people tend to be anxious to please and afraid to offend.

Directly invite people to be honest with you. When they give you negative feedback, don't get defensive. Encourage them to continue. Ask questions: help them clarify their thoughts and be specific in their comments.

You may find people within your organisation — a supervisor, mentor or trusted colleague — who will provide you with feedback. It may also be appropriate, sometimes even necessary, to go outside the organisation and seek feedback from a spouse, friends or an independent consultant.

To get started on this, list your various task areas at work. Then, for each area, identify potential sources of support and possible sources of feedback.

If you have difficulties with receiving support, you will find more detailed advice on this in Chapter 14.

Handling other people at work

Stuart Schmidt and David Kipnis[4] describe six strategies that people commonly use to influence their superiors:

reasoning, confrontation, friendliness, obtaining support from others, gaining the patronage of higher authorities, and bargaining.

Which works best? It appears that people who use confrontation, both men and women, end up with less than those who use reasoning and the other methods. Confronters also experience the highest levels of stress and the lowest levels of job satisfaction.

Many people confuse influence with power. But, as Elaina Zuker[5] points out, power (in the sense of domination) is often the least effective form of influence. There may be short-term gains in pushing others around, but in the long run, power leads to unwilling cooperation rather than mutually beneficial relationships.

Whether manager or employee, you are likely to get more of what you want (and less of what you don't) if you learn how to exercise influence rather than wield power. Sometimes confrontation is necessary, but is best resorted to after all else has been tried. Old-style managers and union leaders would do well to take note! Many of the examples of assertiveness versus aggressiveness (on page 224) apply to the workplace.

There is more advice on handling other people in Chapter 13.

Enhancing workplace effectiveness

Many of the techniques of emotional control and behavioural change described in other parts of this book can benefit you and your workplace in two main ways. First, if you are able to control dysfunctional emotions, you will experience less distress and be free to use your emotional energy more productively. Secondly, you can free up essential workplace skills that may be blocked by self-defeating thinking. Here are some examples:

- *Conflict management.* You can deal with conflict assertively, rather than becoming aggressive or avoidant, once you have removed any blocks to articulating what you want and don't want (see Chapter 13).

- *Time management.* Confronting avoidance and low frustration tolerance will help you manage your workload and get more done (see Chapter 15).

- *Communication skills.* Changing beliefs like: 'I must always look good in front of my colleagues'; 'I must always receive the approval of my superiors'; 'My subordinates must never think badly of me'; and 'I should be able to communicate better' will make it easier for managers and staff to communicate honestly and effectively (see Chapter 14).

- *Delivering performance appraisals.* Self-defeating beliefs, like the ones just listed, will block managers from giving accurate feedback to employees. Skills such as *rational self-analysis* (page 70) can help them address their own high need for approval, overconcern with negative reactions by employees, and self-downing about their management performance.

- *Effective leadership.* Managers who develop flexible attitudes and an adaptive, change-oriented approach to new programmes and ideas are able to motivate and inspire their staff.

- *Creative decision-making.* Creativity is enhanced when internal blocks to change are addressed, especially self-defeating beliefs such as: 'We can't move ahead unless we are sure of success'; 'Profits must always go up'; 'I must always receive positive feedback from my superiors'; or 'My employees must always perceive me as a nice person' (see Chapter 17).

Helping people learn new ways of dealing with their emotions and stress will, in the long run, increase their performance and effectiveness.[6] Perfectionism, for example, paradoxically hinders excellence. Fear of failure or what others will think blocks people from trying their hand at new things. High levels of anxiety slow people down and distract them from problem-solving. Hostility and resentment hinder effective teamwork.

The time put into effectiveness training will be time well spent. It facilitates problem-solving and task completion rather than avoidance. It helps people achieve excellence — and distress-free enjoyment of their work.

The rational principles at work

These benefits are best summed up by showing how the rational principles described in Chapter 5 can be applied to achieve effectiveness in the workplace.

Self-knowledge

- Know what you don't know. Acknowledging your lacks will keep you on the watch for new knowledge to improve your effectiveness.

- Know what you are suited to. A high-energy, risk- and stimulation-loving person will experience distress in a boring, repetitive job; alternatively, a low-energy, safety-conscious person will not cope well in a high-flying position.

- If you are aware of your desires and weaknesses, you will be better able to maintain appropriate and safe boundaries in the workplace.

- Be clear about your limits. Be able to extend yourself, but know when to ease off and avoid any danger of burnout.

Self-acceptance and confidence

- If you accept yourself without self-rating, you will be able to take and use feedback — including constructive criticism — without feeling defensive.

- Confidence in specific abilities will enable you to use these to the maximum to achieve your goals and make yourself marketable to employers.

- Managers who do not need external evidence of their 'worth' will have less difficulty with a 'participation' approach, because they will not fear that it strips them of their power and authority.

Enlightened self-interest

- Make time to be supportive to others, then you will be supported in turn.

- Are you part of a two-career couple? Facilitating your partner's career will make it more likely they will facilitate yours.

- If you are a manager, consultation and power-sharing will be in your interests in the long run. Help staff feel valued and in control of their work situation by being positive in your dealings with them. Emphasise what you want rather than what you don't. Use control only when there is no valid alternative. Avoid angry reactions, and handle complaints in a constructive way. Give, and therefore invite, positive feedback. Acknowledge and reward special efforts. Helping your staff feel in control will keep you in control.

Tolerance for frustration and discomfort

- Accepting critical feedback on your performance is how you will learn and develop, and thereby increase your work satisfaction. View the discomfort involved as unpleasant but tolerable — and worth the gain.

- If you are a manager, accept the realities of your role. You *will* receive criticism from others. You *will* sometimes end up bearing responsibility for other people's mistakes. The smooth functioning of your operation *will* be disrupted from time to time. If you see such happenings as inevitable and uncomfortable, rather than intolerable, you will be better able to take them in your stride.

Long-range enjoyment

- Rapid changes in the marketplace require a focus on the long-term, and confident leadership able to resist pressure for short-term gains.

- Participatory decision-making may take longer than simply issuing orders, but it will save time in the long run when others, through being involved, make a genuine commitment to what is decided and see the job through.

- In the short run, you may prefer to be up-to-date with your paperwork; but diverting some time to supporting your co-workers will benefit you in the long-term.

- Confrontation may seem like the quickest way to get what you want — and sometimes this will be the case — but winning people over with reasoning and friendliness will get you more in the long run.

Risk-taking

- Sometimes businesses do go to the wall, but few would get off the ground in the first place if there was no-one with a vision prepared to take an initial step of faith.

- Choices will not always be black and white. Sometimes you will have to go with the best of the options open to you, without certainty of success. If you have trouble with this, consider the consequences of not making a decision.

Moderation

- To avoid burnout, watch for obsessiveness or over-involvement with your work. Take regular breaks, especially when you feel a compulsion to keep on working. Go home when your colleagues do. Keep your work in balance with the rest of your life.

- Adopt a moderate approach to your dealings with co-workers and subordinates. Reasonableness and negotiation will create a less stressful environment.

- Maintain appropriate boundaries. Be friendly, socialise and share mutual support with co-workers or subordinates, but keep within limits that protect you and them.

Emotional and behavioural responsibility

- Take responsibility for how you feel about your work and how you respond to the treatment you receive. There may be dysfunctional elements to your workplace, but blaming will just keep you a victim — and set you up for burnout.

- Emotional responsibility will reduce the time and energy workers and managers spend on self-defeating reactions to frustrating circumstances; and, instead, help them look for solutions.

Self-direction and commitment

- Workers are more likely to feel distress when they perceive a lack of power in respect of decisions that affect them, they have too much or too little work, there is under- or over-promotion, responsibility is not matched with authority, objectives or requirements are unclear, conflict exists between multiple job demands, or training is inadequate.

Are you unsure what is expected of you in your job? If so, seek clarification of what you are supposed to be achieving. If you lack the necessary training, ask for it or seek it out yourself. Decide what changes to your role you would like, and negotiate on these.

- Self-directed people don't wait for things to happen or other people to do things to them. They see problems and initiate action and change. If they want support, they go and get it. In turn, they watch out for colleagues who may be under extra stress and offer to lend a hand.

- Self-directed people do not feel a need to compete with their peers — they know what they want and work towards getting it, without envying what others are getting. Being non-competitive frees them to enjoy mutually supportive relationships with their colleagues.

Flexibility

Flexibility aids survival in organisations.

- The modern workplace is characterised by significant changes in the composition of the workforce. There are, for example, increasing numbers of women and members of ethnic minorities who bring new values, desires and goals. This requires organisations to be flexible and adaptive, and free of rigid, absolutistic attitudes that interfere with cooperation and problem-solving.

- There is an increasing level of major international competition. Businesses must be more alert than ever to changes in the marketplace and able to respond quickly, or even anticipate them.

- New technology means old ways of doing things may no longer be appropriate. Resistance to change can be costly. It can trigger distress for many people in an organisation, and sometimes even lead to organisational failure. Anticipating change rather than simply waiting for it to happen, as Bartol and Martin have pointed out, can significantly reduce any negative impact it may have.[7]

- Research has found that managers who do not cope well with stress fear change, tend to be inflexible, and lack problem-solving skills. Those who cope better see organisational changes as challenges rather than threats, are highly flexible and adaptable, and are willing to try new ways of dealing with problems.[8] Effective supervisors, rather than dictating procedures and allowing no flexibility, explain the aims of a job and guidelines for achieving these in a general fashion, leaving staff to accomplish the goals in their own way.[9]

Objective thinking

- The modern business setting is not a place for 'magical thinking'. Commercial survival requires that feet be firmly on the ground.

- Make sure you are in touch with reality. Rid yourself especially of any myths about how human beings work. Study psychology. Know, for example, how to get the best out of people by appealing to their enlightened self-interest rather than moralising about what they 'should' do.

Acceptance of reality

Finally, be able to roll with the punches. No matter how well you do as an employee, an executive or the boss, you are unlikely to succeed at everything to which you set your hand. Acceptance of reality will help you to avoid overreacting when things don't work out and, instead of railing against fate, to pick yourself up and start again.

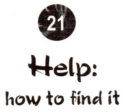

Help:
how to find it

This book has presented a range of skills you can use to minimise unhealthy reactions to stress. Most of them you will be able to learn and use on yourself throughout your life. However, like most other people, from time to time you may face situations that are unfamiliar and beyond your experience. These are the times when it makes sense to ask for help.

Where you can get help

Help may range from informal support given by a friend through to professional therapy for a major difficulty.

Informal support

Most support comes from informal sources such as a partner, friend, relative, neighbour or co-worker. Support may simply involve a listening ear from a neighbour over the fence or advice from a colleague during a coffee break.

Support groups

These are groups where people get together with others who have a similar problem, to share support and advice. Here are some examples of support groups based on specific problems:

- *Physical illness or disability:* support groups for people facing cancer, head injury, arthritis, etc.

- *Negotiating life transitions:* bereavement groups, day centres for the elderly.

- *Addiction:* S.M.A.R.T. Recovery, Alcoholics Anonymous.

- *Mental health:* Schizophrenia Fellowship, GROW, Phobic Trust.

- *Family problems:* Parentline, ToughLove.

Self-help groups that are well run can be very helpful. There is, however, potential for a self-help group to make a problem worse. This can happen when the focus is on whining about a problem rather than dealing with it. When this happens, such groups seek to turn members into 'victims', constantly complaining about injustices done and hindering any attempt to rise above their problems. Fortunately, most support groups are not like this. Just check out a potential group to ensure it is devoted either to developing solutions or to helping people reach acceptance. Talk to others who have had involvement with the group, or attend a session before making up your mind.

Skills training

Skills training is designed to develop ability in areas such as assertiveness and communication. You may get this from an individual counsellor, although it is more usual to do the training in small groups. Such training is often provided by polytechnics, adult education classes or social service organisations.

Professional help

Sometimes professional help is needed, because of the difficulty or complexity of a problem.

- *Counselling* involves such things as giving advice, assisting with decision-making and problem-solving, and may include skills training. It does not assume that the individual needs to change but instead attempts to find solutions to problems.

- *Psychotherapy* assumes that the problem lies mainly within the person, and seeks to help an individual make long-term changes in their typical ways of reacting to life. Psychotherapy is especially relevant to emotional difficulties such as depression and anxiety, and to helping people change self-defeating behaviours such as addiction and violence.

In practice, counselling and psychotherapy are often one and the same. Counselling frequently results in permanent change in an individual; and psychotherapy often needs to be combined with advice-giving or problem-solving.

Traditionally, counselling and psychotherapy have been provided by helping professionals such as psychologists and social workers, but in recent times training courses devoted specifically to counselling or psychotherapy have been available. Do not worry too much about the label a particular helping professional has. Instead, go on recommendations from an adviser you trust or someone who has actually consulted the professional concerned. Here are some of the more common sources of professional help:

- family doctor
- health service social worker or psychologist
- private counsellor/psychotherapist
- Māori health service
- Relationship Services

- alcohol or drug addiction service

- church social service.

Support and crisis services
Sometimes there will be a problem that requires immediate help. Support in a crisis situation can be obtained from services such as Victim Support, Women's Refuge centres, Rape Crisis centres and the Lifeline telephone counselling service.

Where to get advice on sources of help
If you are unsure where to go for help, consider consulting your family doctor, pastor, local Citizens' Advice Bureau, or a local service advertised in your telephone book.

Before you see a counsellor ...

You can increase the chance that counselling or psycho-therapy will be a satisfying experience if you do some advance checking, and monitor your ongoing contact with the counsellor. The following suggestions are adapted from the checklist developed by Stephen Palmer and Kasia Szymanska,[1] as well as from my own experience.

Questions to consider in advance or soon after commencing
- Does the counsellor have relevant qualifications and experience?

- Does the counsellor receive supervision from another professional counsellor or supervision group? (Most professional bodies consider supervision to be mandatory.)

- Is the person a member of a professional body with a code of ethics by which they abide? (Obtain a copy of the code if possible.)

- What type of approach do they use and how does it relate to your problem?

- Discuss your goals and what you expect to get from the counselling.

- Ask about the fees, if any, and discuss the frequency and estimated duration of the sessions.

- Finally, do not enter into a long-term counselling contract unless you are satisfied this is *necessary* and *beneficial* to you. (If in doubt, get a second opinion.)

Points to keep in mind when seeing a counsellor

- *Regular reviews.* Ask for evaluations of progress toward the specified goals.

- *Keep the focus on your problems.* Self-disclosure by the counsellor can sometimes be therapeutically useful, but speak up if the sessions are dominated by the counsellor discussing their own problems at length.

- *Maintain appropriate boundaries between yourself and your counsellor.* Do not accept significant gifts (apart from relevant therapeutic material, such as reading) or social invitations (unless they are part of the therapeutic work itself — like, for instance, facing social anxiety by going with your counsellor to a crowded coffee bar). If your counsellor proposes a change in venue for the counselling sessions — for example, from a centre to the counsellor's own home — without good reason, do not agree. It is not beneficial (in fact, it is usually damaging) for clients to have sexual contact with their counsellor, and it is unethical for counsellors or therapists to engage in any such contact with their clients.

- *Express any concerns.* If at any time you feel discounted, undermined or manipulated, or have any doubts about the counselling you are receiving, discuss this with your counsellor. Try to resolve issues as they arise rather than sit on them. If you are still uncertain, seek advice. Talk to a friend, your doctor, local Citizens' Advice Bureau, local Advocacy Service, the professional body to which your counsellor belongs, or the agency (if any) that employs them.

Overcoming the blocks to asking for help

I doubt that change is possible

If you don't see much chance of anything changing, you will probably let things drift. Use the principle of *objective thinking* (page 65) to overcome inertia:

- Challenge any myths about accepting help. How do you know that change is impossible until you have given it a try?

- Dispute any 'magical thinking' that your emotions are controlled or your life mapped out by external forces.

I might end up dependent on someone else

Do you believe that people should not need help with personal problems and should be able to 'stand on their own feet' or that to accept help would somehow be proof of 'weakness'? Do you worry that if you seek help from other people you will become dependent on them?

- Review the principles of *self-acceptance and confidence* (page 58). Asking for help does not show you are a 'weak person' — all it proves is that you are a person who sometimes requires assistance.

- Trust your own judgements about the advice you get — decide which parts are right for you, and leave the rest.

- Know what your limits are. Know how far you can go with helping yourself, and when it is time to use other people for support and guidance.

- Keep in mind the principle of *emotional and behavioural responsibility* (page 63). Remember that you create your own emotions and behaviours, and only you can change them. Other people can show you what to do, but only you can do it. If you keep that in mind, you are unlikely to become dependent.

I might lose control to someone else

Do you worry that you will be made to do things against your will, such as adopting beliefs which are against your values? Apply the principle of *self-direction* (page 63):

- Take from others what will work for you, and leave the rest.

- If you sense that a helper is trying to force something on you, discuss it with them. If they don't listen, exercise your choice to go elsewhere.

It's too dangerous to reveal yourself to others

Do you fear that the counsellor will regard you as insane, or that you will end up with a formal psychiatric diagnosis? Do you think that if you expose your thoughts and feelings to another person they will use what they learn to harm you, get power over you, or at the very least look down on you? *Risk-taking* (page 62) and *self-acceptance* (page 58) are key principles that will help you overcome these fears.

- There are some risks in accepting help. Sometimes people do inappropriately use what they know. Sometimes they do look down on others. But keep in mind three questions: Just how damaging would these things be if they did happen? How likely are they to happen? And is the risk worth it — in comparison to the potential gain (or the certainty of staying where you are if you do nothing)?

- As you move from self-evaluation to self-acceptance, you will become less concerned about what other people may think when you expose your thoughts and feelings to them.

Changing is too scary

Most people would not consciously resist getting better, but sometimes there are secondary gains from staying as they are. Getting attention through being ill is an example. Probably the main motivation is avoidance of responsibility: if a person learns to handle stress, they lose a useful justification for avoiding life's problems, difficulties and challenges.

- Re-study the principle of *tolerance for frustration and discomfort* (page 61). If you accept discomfort as a normal part of life and believe that facing it is in your interests, you will feel easier about seeking help and beginning the process of personal change.

- Practise *flexibility* (page 64). Be open to exploring new ways of looking at yourself, others, the world, and life in general. Opening up new vistas and helping people change is the essence of counselling and psychotherapy.

Be realistic about change

Finally, watch for any internal demand that you be able to change anything and everything you dislike. This may lead to potentially dangerous behaviour — like, for example, radical dieting — and, finally to disillusionment. The principle of *acceptance* (page 65) will help you avoid these dangers while still working hard at change. Go for help with optimism and a determination to achieve the change you want. Keep in mind, however, that you can't change everything.[2] How do you strive for change while at the same time accepting its limitations? The answer is to desire change — but keep your desire as a preference, not a demand.

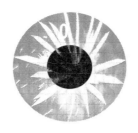

Extras

Life control options questionnaire

Step one

Begin by answering the questions on the following pages. Don't think about how you will answer any of the questions for very long — write down your response to each item quickly. Be honest: make sure you put down what you really think about the item (not what you believe you are supposed to think). Use the following scoring system:

Doesn't really apply to me	Moderate or happens sometimes	Significant or happens frequently
leave blank	**1**	**2**

Write your answers in the box beside each number. Ignore the numbers in the right-hand column for now.

1	☐	I have trouble saying 'no' when people ask things of me	5
2	☐	I eat the wrong things	7
3	☐	I don't have much to do with friends and acquaintances	4
4	☐	I have a trembling feeling	13
5	☐	I don't have a regular pattern of going to bed and getting up in the morning	9
6	☐	I get into arguments with my partner that are not resolved	6
7	☐	I have thought that maybe I had better cut down on my drinking	10
8	☐	I find it hard to think up alternative ways to solve problems	3
9	☐	I have difficulty swallowing, get wind, make indigestion noises	7
10	☐	I get annoyed when someone comments on my use of alcohol	10
11	☐	I have difficulty making decisions about everyday matters	1
12	☐	I find it hard to control my eating	11
13	☐	I suffer stomach pain, a burning sensation, feeling of fullness, nausea, vomiting	7
14	☐	I get breathless	13
15	☐	I hate to think that I might be a burden to others	5
16	☐	I have to think hard when confronted with a moral dilemma	1
17	☐	I feel little affection for my partner	6
18	☐	I don't attend club or social activities	4, 12
19	☐	I tend to take on too many tasks or commitments at once	1, 14
20	☐	I often put off doing anything about problems	3
21	☐	I wish that my partner and I spent more quality time together	6
22	☐	I get confronted with problems which seem unsolvable	3
23	☐	I don't eat at least one hot, balanced meal in a day	7
24	☐	I don't get 7–8 hours sleep at least four times a week	9
25	☐	I feel physically unfit	8
26	☐	My sleep is unsatisfying	9
27	☐	I suffer from constipation	7, 8
28	☐	It seems as though everything goes wrong at once for me	3
29	☐	I use drugs that are not prescribed by a doctor in order to change my mood	11
30	☐	I get pains or a feeling of pressure or constriction in my chest	13

31	☐	I have a drink first thing in the morning to steady my nerves or get rid of a hangover	10
32	☐	My sleep is broken	9
33	☐	I feel overwhelmed when confronted with more than one problem at a time	3
34	☐	I perform poorly at work, find it hard to make decisions, forget things, put off important work	14
35	☐	My blood pressure tends to be high	13
36	☐	I drink more than six cups of tea or coffee in a day	11
37	☐	I suffer from headaches or other pain, often in the neck or lower back	13
38	☐	I worry about making others feel bad	5
39	☐	I tend to put off making decisions	1, 2
40	☐	I'm not happy in my relationship with my partner	6
41	☐	I over-comply by rigidly applying rules and instructions	14
42	☐	I feel compelled to gamble	11
43	☐	I tend to panic when confronted with a difficult problem	3
44	☐	At work, I tend to over-identify with consumers/customers	14
45	☐	I worry about making wrong decisions in case there are unpleasant results	1
46	☐	I feel a compulsion to exercise which I find hard to control	11
47	☐	I often don't know what to say to people	4
48	☐	I worry about weight but do nothing about it	7, 8
49	☐	I take tranquillisers	11
50	☐	I don't confide in one or more friends about personal matters	4
51	☐	I don't tend to give and receive affection	4
52	☐	I have been in trouble with the law because of alcohol	10
53	☐	I have so much to do there's not much time for rest or personal relationships	1, 2
54	☐	I don't communicate much with the people I live with about domestic issues	4
55	☐	I wake early in the morning and can't get back to sleep	9
56	☐	I feel guilty if I put what I want ahead of what others want	5
57	☐	I don't really know what my overall goals in life are	1
58	☐	I have feelings of tension, am overly alert/keyed up/easily startled	13

59	☐	I feel guilty about my drinking	10
60	☐	I don't take quiet time for myself during the day	12
61	☐	I find it hard to ask other people for what I want	5
62	☐	I don't take lunch or tea breaks, avoid my colleagues	12, 14
63	☐	I don't take holidays	1, 12, 14
64	☐	I take work home	2
65	☐	I find it hard to get motivated to do things	8
66	☐	My weight is not right for my height	8
67	☐	I feel fatigued when I wake up in the morning	9
68	☐	I can't seem to change how I react to problems even though my behaviour is unhelpful	3
69	☐	I am not coping well with my job; at times I am inefficient, slow, rude, forgetful, miss days	2
70	☐	I find it hard to fall asleep	8, 9, 12
71	☐	My home life is stressful	6
72	☐	At work, I feel resentment towards the customers/consumers	14
73	☐	I am restless, can't relax	13
74	☐	I don't exercise vigorously	8
75	☐	I take sleeping tablets	9, 11
76	☐	I don't seem to organise my time effectively	2
77	☐	I find it hard to confront other people when I'm unhappy with their actions	5
78	☐	I have a negative attitude toward my workplace; frequently complain and blame others	14
79	☐	My heart beats rapidly	13
80	☐	I feel like leaving my partner	6
81	☐	I stay late, work excessive overtime, think about my job when not at work	12, 14
82	☐	I put off doing things	2
83	☐	I miss deadlines	2
84	☐	I experience looseness of bowels	7
85	☐	Friends and relatives have said that I am not a normal drinker	10
86	☐	I get tired more easily than I used to	8

87	☐	I feel used by other people	5
88	☐	My partner and I don't communicate well	6
89	☐	I rush lunch	12, 14
90	☐	I tend to bottle up strong emotions like anger or worry rather than talk them out	4
91	☐	I overeat beyond the point of comfort	7
92	☐	I tend to avoid saying what I think if there's a chance others may disagree with me	5
93	☐	My partner, parent or another near relative complains about my drinking	10
94	☐	I smoke	11
95	☐	When I try to solve problems I tend to make things worse	3
96	☐	I don't do things for fun	12
97	☐	I drink to the point where I am affected by alcohol	10
98	☐	The sexual relationship with my partner is unsatisfying	6
99	☐	I get home late from work	2
100	☐	I feel shy in social situations	4

Step two

Transfer your answers to the scoring box (on the next page). Using the numbers in the right-hand column of the question list as a guide, transfer your '1's and '2's to the space (headed 'SCORES') alongside the corresponding number in the scoring box. For example, let's say that for question 1 you wrote '2' — you would then put a '2' alongside item 5 in the scoring box. If for question 2 you wrote '1', you would then put a '1' alongside item 7 in the scoring box. If there are two (or more) numbers in the right-hand column, put a score for each. For example, if for question 20 you put a '1', you would then put a '1' alongside both of items 4 and 12 in the scoring box.

Add up the numbers for each item in the scoring box and write the total in the TOTALS column. Then transfer the totals to the **Alternatives for Action** sheet (on the following page), circling the appropriate number in each case. These scores indicate the extent to which pursuing each action choice might be helpful for you.

	SCORES	TOTALS
1		
2		
3		
4		
5		
6		
7		
8		
9		
10		
11		
12		
13		
14		

Alternatives for Action

Put a circle round the (nearest) number which applies to each item.

1 2 3 4 5 6 7 8 9 10 11 12 13 14 15 16								**1**	Clarify my goals so that I know where I'm going (Chap. 12).
1 2 3 4 5 6 7 8 9 10 11 12 13 14 15 16								**2**	Increase my skills for managing time so that I get more done (Chap. 15).
1 2 3 4 5 6 7 8 9 10 11 12 13 14 15 16								**3**	Improve my problem-solving skills (Chap. 19).
1 2 3 4 5 6 7 8 9 10 11 12 13 14 15 16								**4**	Develop a support system and enhance communication (Chap. 14).
1 2 3 4 5 6 7 8 9 10 11 12 13 14 15 16								**5**	Extend my range of assertiveness skills (Chap. 13).
1 2 3 4 5 6 7 8 9 10 11 12 13 14 15 16								**6**	Develop my personal relationships so that they are more satisfying (Chap. 14).
1 2 3 4 5 6 7 8 9 10 11 12 13 14 15 16								**7**	Upgrade to a diet that helps me feel good in the long term (Chap. 9).
1 2 3 4 5 6 7 8 9 10 11 12 13 14 15 16								**8**	Change my exercise programme to achieve long-term gain (Chap. 9).
1 2 3 4 5 6 7 8 9 10 11 12 13 14 15 16								**9**	Institute a programme to help me sleep better (Chap. 11).
1 2 3 4 5 6 7 8 9 10 11 12 13 14 15 16								**10**	Moderate my alcohol use so I can enjoy it in the long-term (Chap. 9).

1	2	3	4	5	6	7	8	**11**	Change other addictive behaviour from short- to long-term gain (Chap. 9).
9	10	11	12	13	14	15	16		
1	2	3	4	5	6	7	8	**12**	Take time to do what I want and improve efficiency at work (Chap. 15).
9	10	11	12	13	14	15	16		
1	2	3	4	5	6	7	8	**13**	Develop skills to let go of tension (Chap. 10).
9	10	11	12	13	14	15	16		
1	2	3	4	5	6	7	8	**14**	Modify some work habits to avoid risk of burnout (Chap. 20).
9	10	11	12	13	14	15	16		

Interpreting your scores

The higher your score for any particular item, the more likely you are to benefit from doing some work in that area. Note that a high score for any one item does not mean that work on that area is an absolute 'necessity'; rather, it will help you identify where, out of all the areas you could work on, your time might be best spent.

Sleep log

Week beginning: ....

Fill out this sleep log every morning as soon as possible after getting up. Guess the approximate times (your figures do not have to be absolutely correct). To calculate averages for the week, add up the figures then divide by 7.

Day								Ave
Total minutes spent napping yesterday								
If any sleeping medication taken, show amount and time taken								
Time you turned out your lights intending to try to sleep								
Number of minutes it took you to first fall asleep last night								
If you woke during the night, number of minutes you were awake								
Number of times you woke last night								
Number of hours you slept last night								
When was the last time you woke up this morning?								
When did you get out of bed for the last time this morning?								
Total number of hours you were in bed last night								
By your own average, how well did you sleep last night? *Choose from list A below.*								
Generally speaking, how well did you sleep last night? *Choose from list B below.*								
Overall, how refreshing was your sleep? *Choose one from list C below.*								

Compared with my usual average *for the past month*, I slept:

A

1. Much worse.
2. A bit worse.
3. About average.
4. A bit better.
5. Much better.

B

1. About the worst night's sleep I could imagine.
2. Poor sleep.
3. Fair sleep, but still not satisfactory.
4. Good sleep — but with some disturbance.
5. Excellent sleep.

C

1. I got no refreshment at all from the time I spent in bed.
2. Slightly refreshing.
3. Refreshing, but still not really adequate.
4. Fairly refreshing.
5. Completely refreshing.

Adapted from: Sloan E.P., Hauri P., Bootzin R., Morin C., Stevenson M., & Shapiro, C.M. (1993). The Nuts and Bolts of Behavioral Therapy for Insomnia. *Journal of Psychosomatic Research*, Vol. 37, Suppl. 1, pp. 19–37.

Sleep questionnaire

If you have trouble sleeping, this questionnaire will help you identify the causes. As you go through the questionnaire, tick any boxes that apply to you.

Sleep environment

☐ Noise   ☐ Too warm

☐ Shift work   ☐ Too cool

☐ Time-zone changes   ☐ Uncomfortable bed

☐ Bed-partner restless or noisy or snores

☐ Other ....
....

Sleep routine

☐ Heavy meal close to bedtime   ☐ Read or watch television in bed

☐ Little exercise during the day   ☐ Tense while lying in bed

☐ Exercise close to bedtime   ☐ Bed is uncomfortable

☐ Irregular times for going to bed and getting up   ☐ Work in bed or in your bedroom

☐ Hard to switch off your mind when you go to bed

☐ Other ....
....

Substance use

☐ Prescribed sleeping pills   ☐ Cold remedies

☐ Over-the-counter sleep aids   ☐ Appetite suppressants

☐ Tranquillisers   ☐ Stimulants

☐ Diuretic or water-reducing medication   ☐ Slimming pills

☐ Nicotine: ...... cigarettes/cigars/pipes per day

☐ Drugs such as heroin, cocaine, cannabis, amphetamines, LSD or other hallucinogens:

....
....

☐ Caffeine: .... cups of tea, coffee or other caffeinated drinks per day, last cup at .... pm

☐ Other fluids: .... cups/glasses in evening, last at .... pm

☐ Chocolate: .... during the day, last used at .... pm

☐ Alcohol: .... standard drinks per day, last drink at .... pm

(standard drink = 200 ml beer, small glass of wine, one measure of spirits).

Physical health

☐ Pain

☐ Heart problems

☐ Breathing problems

☐ Emphysema

☐ Asthma

☐ Hiatus hernia

☐ Enlarged prostate

☐ Stomach and digestive disorders

☐ High blood pressure

☐ Other ....
....

☐ Cancer

☐ Kidney failure

☐ Parkinson's disease

☐ Starvation (including anorexia)

☐ Food allergies

☐ Significantly over- or under-weight

☐ Cough

☐ Toothache

☐ Arthritis

Emotions

☐ Anxiety/worrying

☐ Panic attacks

☐ Anger

☐ Other ....
....

☐ Depression

☐ Stress

☐ Guilt

Miscellaneous symptoms

☐ You wake in the early morning hours and cannot get back to sleep at all, no matter what you do

☐ You uncontrollably fall asleep at odd times during the day, for either a few seconds or for longer periods

☐ After feeling a strong emotion (such as laughter, anger or surprise) your muscles feel very weak

☐ Just before going to sleep and just after you wake you are unable to move or speak

☐ At the point where you are falling asleep or waking up, you experience vivid, dream-like images

☐ You have a restless, uncomfortable feeling in the legs that you can relieve only by moving or stimulating the legs, for instance by walking around

While asleep, you experience:

☐ Frequent leg or arm jerks, or general thrashing around

☐ Snoring

☐ Irregular breathing or gasping for breath

☐ Intense anxiety (not associated with any dream) which leads you to cry out (as an adult)

☐ Sleepwalking (as an adult)

Beliefs about sleep

Listed below are a number of statements reflecting beliefs and attitudes about sleep. Indicate to what extent you personally agree or disagree with each statement, using this scale.

Strongly disagree	Disagree	Unsure	Agree	Strongly agree
1	2	3	4	5

☐ Going for one or two nights without sleep will inevitably have serious consequences

☐ Chronic insomnia will lead to a nervous breakdown

☐ If I spend more time in bed I can get more sleep and feel better the next day

☐ When it is hard to sleep, the best thing is to stay in bed and keep trying

☐ If I have a poor night's sleep, I won't be able to function the next day

☐ It is better to take a sleeping pill than have a poor night's sleep

☐ There is nothing wrong with using sleeping pills on a permanent basis

☐ Everyone needs eight hours of sleep

☐ Insomnia is the result of ageing and there isn't much can be done about it

☐ Feeling bad or not functioning well is mostly caused by not sleeping well

☐ Insomnia is mainly caused by biochemical factors in the body

☐ Alcohol before bedtime is a good way to get a night's sleep

☐ I must be able to feel and function at my best every day, which requires a good night's sleep

- [ ] There is little I can do to handle the tiredness, irritability, anxiety and poor functioning that results from poor sleep
- [ ] It is awful to have a sleepless night and I can't stand the way I feel the next day
- [ ] I absolutely must get a good sleep every night
- [ ] I should be able to sleep well every night, no matter where I am or what is happening in my life
- [ ] Insomnia is ruining my ability to enjoy life and stopping me from achieving my goals

Assertiveness questionnaire

The following questionnaire will help you identify any unassertive tendencies. Assign a score to each question, using this rating scale:

I do this most of the time	I do this fairly often	I do this half the time	I do this now and again	I hardly ever do this
1	2	3	4	5

Doormat behaviour

- **1**   I want something but fail to ask for it
- **2**   I say nothing when someone behaves in a way I dislike
- **3**   I do something I do not wish to do, or which is highly inconvenient for me
- **4**   I modify my speech and behaviour to conform to those around me
- **5**   I ask permission of others before I do or say things
- **6**   I apologise for things even when I am not responsible

Holding in emotions

- **7**   I tell myself it is wrong to feel angry towards another person
- **8**   When I am annoyed, I hold it in rather than express it
- **9**   When someone is behaving toward me in a way I dislike, I get very tense in my body
- **10**   I feel resentful because I believe I am being forced to do something or deprived of what I want

Aggressiveness

- **11**   I ignore the interests of others in what I do and say
- **12**   I blame and accuse others when things go wrong
- **13**   I threaten others to get them to cooperate with me
- **14**   I feel hostile toward others and try to get back at them

Calculate your scores for each section as follows:

- Add your answers to numbers 1 to 6 here: . . . . ,

  then divide this total by 6: . . . .

  (this is your *doormat behaviour* score).

- Add your answers to numbers 7 to 10 here: . . . . ,

  then divide this total by 4: . . . .

  (this is your *holding in emotions* score).

- Add your answers to numbers 11 to 14 here: . . . . ,

  then divide this total by 4: . . . .

  (this is your *aggressive behaviour* score).

A score of 3 indicates this may be a problem; 4 or 5 suggests that some work on that area is a priority.

Time control questionnaire

Score each item as follows:

Never	Occasionally	Often	Almost all the time
0	1	2	3

☐ I think that I have used my time poorly.

☐ It seems like I am working under constant pressure.

☐ It seems there are not enough hours in the day.

☐ I feel overloaded.

☐ I feel frustrated because I am not able to finish the jobs I regard as important.

☐ I find myself doing things I don't want to do.

☐ I spend evenings and weekends working to meet deadlines.

☐ I miss deadlines.

☐ I find it hard to trust subordinates with tasks, so I do them myself.

☐ I have trouble making decisions about what to do.

☐ I tend to lack time for personal relationships, rest and recreation.

..... Add up your scores.

How to interpret your total score:

0–11:   You are probably controlling your time reasonably well.

12–22:   Some work on your time control would be useful.

23–33:   You would be wise to make time control a priority.

Make a note of the specific items on which you scored higher, so you can give them particular attention.

Professional books and articles on personal control & stress management

The literature in this section will primarily be of interest to helping professionals offering stress management counselling and providing consultancy to workplace organisations. Some items may also be of interest to the general public.

The causes of stress

Gribbin, John, and Gribben, Mary. (1993). *Being Human: Putting people in an evolutionary perspective*. London: J.M. Dent.

Palmer, Stephen. (1992). *Stress Management: A course reader*. London: Centre for Stress Management.

Toates, F. (1988). *Biological foundations of behaviour*. Milton Keynes: Open University.

Thinking and stress

DiGiuseppe, Raymond. (1996). The Nature of Irrational and Rational Beliefs: Progress in Rational Emotive Behaviour Therapy. *Journal of Rational-Emotive and Cognitive-Behaviour Therapy,* 14:1, 5–28.

Himle, David P. (1989). Changing Personal Rules. *Journal of Rational-Emotive and Cognitive-Behaviour Therapy*, 7:2, 79–92.

Ruth, William J. (1992). Irrational Thinking in Humans: An evolutionary proposal for Ellis' genetic postulate. *Journal of Rational-Emotive and Cognitive-Behaviour Therapy*, 10:1, 3–20.

Low discomfort/frustration-tolerance

Ellis, Albert. (1986). Discomfort Anxiety: A new cognitive behavioral construct. In Ellis, A., and Greiger, R. (eds). *Handbook Of Rational-Emotive Therapy (Vol 2)*. New York: Springer.

Ellis, Albert. (1987). A Sadly Neglected Cognitive Element in Depression. *Cognitive Therapy and Research*, 11, 121–146.

Ellis, Albert. (2003). Discomfort Anxiety: A new cognitive-behavioral construct. *Journal of Rational-Emotive and Cognitive-Behaviour Therapy*, 21:3/4, 183–202.

Froggatt, W. (2002). *The Rational Treatment of Anxiety: An outline for cognitive-behavioural intervention with clinical anxiety disorders*. Hastings: Rational Training Resources.

Rational Effectiveness Training

Anderson, J.P. (2002). Executive Coaching: Some comments from the field. *Journal of Rational-Emotive and Cognitive-Behaviour Therapy*, 20:3/4, 223–234.

Cooper, C., and Cartwright, S. (1996). *Mental Health and Stress in the Workplace: A guide for employers*. London: HMSO.

DiMattia, D., and Ijzermans, T. (1996). *Reaching Their Minds: A trainer's manual for rational effectiveness training*. New York: Institute for Rational-Emotive Therapy.

Dryden, W. (1990). *Creativity in Rational-Emotive Therapy*. Loughton, Essex: Gale Centre Publications.

Ellis, Albert, and DiMattia, Dominic. (1991). *Rational Effectiveness Training: A new method of facilitating management and labor relations*. New York: Institute for Rational-Emotive Therapy.

Ellis, A., Gordon, J., Neenan, M., and Palmer, S. (1997). *Stress Counselling: A rational emotive behavioural approach*. London: Cassell.

Forman, S.G., and Forman, B.D. (1980). Rational-Emotive Staff Development. *Psychology in the Schools*, 17, 90–96.

France, R., and Robson, M. (1997). *Cognitive Behavioural Therapy in Primary Care*. London: Jessica Kingsley.

Johnson, B.W., Huwe, J.M., and Lucas, J.L. (2000). Rational Mentoring. *Journal of Rational-Emotive and Cognitive-Behavior Therapy*, 18:1, 39–54.

Klarreich, S.H., DiGuiseppe, R., and DiMattia, D. (1987). EAPs: Mind Over Myths. *Personnel Administrator*, 32:2, 119–121.

Kodish, S.P. (2002). Rational Emotive Behaviour Coaching. *Journal of Rational-Emotive and Cognitive-Behaviour Therapy*, 20:3/4, 235–246.

Misc. (2004). Perfectionism: Special Issue of Journal of Rational-Emotive and Cognitive-Behaviour Therapy. *Journal of Rational-Emotive and Cognitive-Behaviour Therapy*, 22:4.

Neenan, Michael. (1993). Rational-Emotive Therapy at Work. *Stress News*, 5:1, 7–10.

Palmer, S., and Dryden, W. (1991). A Multimodal Approach to Stress Management. *Stress News*, 3:1, 2–10.

Palmer, S., Ellis, A., Gordon, J., and Neenan, M. (1998). Group Stress Counselling. *The Rational Emotive Behaviour Therapist*, 6:1, 4–17.

Palmer. S. (2002). Cognitive and Organisational Models of Stress that are Suitable for Use within Workplace Stress Management/Prevention, Coaching, Training and Counselling Settings. *The Rational Emotive Behaviour Therapist*, 10:1, 15–21.

Richman, D.R. (Guest Editor). (1992). Working Together: Belief systems of individuals and organisations. *Journal of Cognitive Psychotherapy*, 6:4, 231–244.

Walen, Susan R., DiGiuseppe, Ray, and Dryden, Windy. (1992). *A Practitioner's Guide To Rational-Emotive Therapy* (2nd edn). New York: Oxford University Press.

Healthy living

Egger, Gary, and Swinburn, Boyd. (1996). *The Fat Loss Handbook: A guide for professionals.* Sydney: Allen and Unwin.

Goleman, Daniel, and Gurin, Joel (eds) (1993). *Mind/Body Medicine.* New York: Consumer Reports Books.

Moorey, Stirling, and Greer, D. (2002). *Cognitive Behaviour Therapy for People With Cancer* (2nd edn). Oxford: Oxford University Press.

White, C.A. (2001). *Cognitive Behavior Therapy for Chronic Medical Problems: A guide to assessment and treatment in practice.* Chichester: Wiley.

Relaxation training

Goldfried, M.R., and Davison, G.C. (1976). *Clinical Behaviour Therapy*. New York: Holt, Rinehart and Winston.

Palmer, Stephen. (1992). *Stress Management: A course reader*. London: Centre for Stress Management.

Sleep problems

Froggatt, W. (2002). *The Rational Treatment of Anxiety: An outline for cognitive-behavioural intervention with clinical anxiety disorders*. Hastings: Rational Training Resources.

Laidlaw, K., Thompson, L.W., Dick-Siskin, L., and Gallagher-Thompson, D. (2003). *Cognitive Behaviour Therapy with Older People*. Chichester: John Wiley.

Morin C.M., Kowatch R.A., Barry T., and Walton E. (1993). Cognitive-Behavior Therapy for Late-Life Insomnia. *Journal of Consulting and Clinical Psychology*, 61:1, 137–46.

Nathan, P., and Gorman, J. (1998). *A Guide to Treatments that Work*. New York: Oxford University Press.

Sloan E.P., Hauri P., Bootzin R., Morin C., Stevenson M., and Shapiro, C.M. (1993). The Nuts and Bolts of Behavioral Therapy for Insomnia. *Journal of Psychosomatic Research*, 37: Suppl. 1, 19–37.

Assertiveness

Carmody, T.P. (1978). Rational-Emotive, Self-Instructional, and Behavioral Assertion Training: Facilitation Maintenance. *Cognitive Therapy and Research*, 2, 241–253.

Lange, A., and Jakubowski, P. (1976). *Responsible Assertive Behaviour: Cognitive-behavioural procedures for trainers*. Champaign, Ill: Research Press.

Robb, Harold B. (1992). Why You Don't Have a 'Perfect Right' to Anything. *Journal of Rational-Emotive and Cognitive-Behavior Therapy*, 10:4, 259–269.

Treatment Protocol Project. (1997). *Management of Mental Disorders* (2nd edn). Sydney: World Health Organization.

Wolfe, J.L., and Fodor, I.G. (1975). A Cognitive-Behavioral Approach to Modifying Assertive Behavior in Women. *Counselling Psychologist*, 5:4, 45–52.

Managing change

Bartol, K. M., and Martin, D. C. (1991). *Management*. New York: McGraw-Hill.

Brown, D. (1990). *Managing for Change: A '90s approach to people resource management in New Zealand*. Auckland: David Bateman.

Di Mattia, et al. (1993). Special Issue: RET in the workplace — Part II. *Journal of Rational-Emotive and Cognitive-Behavior Therapy*, 11:2.

Dryden, W., and Hill, L.K. (eds). (1993). *Innovations in Rational-Emotive Therapy*. London: Sage.

Golzen, G. (1988). *Career Counselling for Executives: A guide to selecting outplacement, redeployment and career management services*. London: Kogan Page.

Palmer, Stephen. (1992). *Stress Management: A course reader*. London: Centre for Stress Management.

Seeking help

Palmer, Stephen, and Szymanska, Kasia. (1994). A Checklist for Clients Interested in Receiving Counselling, Psychotherapy or Hypnosis. *The Rational Emotive Behaviour Therapist*, 2:1, 25–27.

Workplace stress

Cayer, M., DiMattia, D., and Wingrove, J. (1988). Conquering Evaluation Fear. *Personnel Administrator*, 33:6, 97–107.

Cooper, C., and Cartwright, S. 1996. *Mental Health and Stress in the Workplace: A guide for employers*. London: HMSO.

DiMattia, D. (1986). A 'Fast Track' Counselling Approach for EAPs. *Benefits Today*, Nov.

DiMattia, D., Yeager, R., and Dube, I. (1989). Emotional Barriers to Learning. *Personnel Journal*, 68:11, 86–89.

European Agency for Safety and Health at Work. (2000). *Research on Work-related Stress*. Luxembourg: Office for Official Publications of the European Communities.

European Agency for Safety and Health at Work. (2002). *Prevention of Psychosocial Risks and Stress at Work in Practice*. Luxembourg: Office for Official Publications of the European Communities.

European Commission. (2002). *How to Tackle Psychosocial Issues and Reduce Work-related Stress*. Luxembourg: Office for Official Publications of the European Communities.

Klarreich, S.H., DiGuiseppe, R., and DiMattia, D. (1987). EAPs: Mind Over Myths. *Personnel Administrator*, 32:2, 119–121.

Palmer. S. (2002). Cognitive and Organisational Models of Stress that are Suitable for Use within Workplace Stress Management/Prevention, Coaching, Training and Counselling Settings. *The Rational Emotive Behaviour Therapist*, 10:1, 15–21.

Richman, D.R. (guest ed). (1992). Working Together: Belief systems of individuals and organisations. *Journal of Cognitive Psychotherapy*, 6:4, 231–244.

Endnotes

Chapter 1

1. Ellis, A. (1994). *Reason and Emotion in Psychotherapy.* (rev edn). New York: Carol Publishing Group.
2. Selye, Hans. (1974). *Stress Without Distress.* London: Hodder & Stoughton.

Chapter 2

1. Freudenberger, H.J. (1980). *Burnout: The high cost of achievement.* New York: Doubleday.
2. American Psychiatric Association. (1994). *Diagnostic and Statistical Manual of Mental Disorders, 4th Edition.* Washington, DC.
3. Froggatt, W. (2003). *FearLess: Your guide to overcoming anxiety.* Auckland: HarperCollins.

Chapter 3

1. Cloninger, C.R., Svrakic, D.M. & Przybek, T.R. (1993). A Psychobiological Model of Temperament and Character. *Archives of General Psychiatry*, 50, 975–990; and Gregson, Olga & Looker, Terry. (1994). The Biological Basis of Stress Management. *British Journal of Guidance and Counselling*, 22:1, 13–26.
2. Bernard, Michael. (1991). *Staying Rational in an Irrational World.* New York: Lyle Stuart.
3. Gregson, Olga & Looker, Terry. (1994). The Biological Basis of Stress Management. *British Journal of Guidance and Counselling*, 22:1, 13–26.
4. Booth-Kewley, S. & Friedman, H.S. (1987). Psychological Predictors of Heart Disease: A quantitative review. *Psychological Bulletin*, 101, 343–362.
5. See Peele, Stanton & DeGrandpre, Richard. (1995). My Genes Made Me Do It. *Psychology Today*, 28:4, 50.

6. Rotter, Julian. (1966). Generalized Expectancies for Internal Versus External Control of Reinforcement. *Psychological Monographs*, 80:1, (Whole No. 609).
7. Asbell, Bernard. (1991). *What They Know About You.* New York: Random House.
8. Ellis, A., McInerney, J., DiGiuseppe, R. & Yeager, R. (1988). *Rational-Emotive Therapy with Alcoholics and Substance Abusers.* Boston: Allyn and Bacon.

Chapter 5

1. Hauck, P.A. (1992). *Overcoming the Rating Game: Beyond self-love — beyond self-esteem.* Louisville, KY: Westminster/ John Knox.
2. Kobasa, Suzanne C. (1979). Stressful Life Events, Personality, and Health: An inquiry into hardiness. *Journal of Personality and Social Psychology*, 37:1, 1–11.
3. A saying originally coined by a Taoist monk, popularised by Reinhold Niebuhr, adopted by Alcoholics Anonymous, paraphrased by Gunars Neiders in *The Conquest of Happiness: A rational approach* (found on the Internet at http://www.halcyon.com/neiders/conquest/conquest.htm), and further paraphrased by this author.

Chapter 6

1. DiMattia, Dominic & Ijzermans, Theo. (1996). *Reaching Their Minds: A trainer's manual for rational effectiveness training.* New York: Institute for Rational-Emotive Therapy.
2. Froggatt, W. (2003). *Choose to be Happy: Your step-by-step guide.* Auckland: HarperCollins.
3. A good selection of tapes is obtainable from the Albert Ellis Institute, 45 East 65th Street, New York 10021-6593, United States of America, Fax 001-212-249-3582, Phone 001-212-535-0822. Internet: http://www.rebt.org/
4. Froggatt, W. (2003). *FearLess: Your guide to overcoming anxiety.* Auckland: HarperCollins.

Chapter 7

1. Froggatt, W. (2003). *FearLess: Your guide to overcoming anxiety.* Auckland: HarperCollins.
2. For a more detailed discussion of perfectionism and how to deal with it, see the chapter on that topic in: Froggatt, Wayne (2003). *Choose to be Happy: Your step-by-step guide.* Auckland: HarperCollins.

Chapter 8

1. Ellis, A. (1971). *Growth Through Reason.* Hollywood: Wilshire Book Co.
2. The procedure of *rational self-analysis* is described in Chapter 6.
3. See Froggatt, W. (2003). *FearLess: Your guide to overcoming anxiety.* Auckland: HarperCollins.
4. This process is adapted from the work of Raymond Novaco: Novaco, R. (1975). *Anger Control.* Lexington, MS: Lexington Books.

Chapter 9

1. US Department of Health and Human Services. (1995). *Dietary Guidelines for Americans.* Washington, DC: US Department of Health and Human Services.
2. King, Olwyn. (1993). *Good For You: The latest word on what to eat.* Petone: Dietwise Publications.

Chapter 10

1. Goldfried, M.R. & Davison, G.C. (1976). *Clinical Behaviour Therapy.* New York: Holt, Rinehart and Winston.

Chapter 11

1. Morin, C.M., Kowatch, R.A., Barry, T. & Walton, E. (1993). Cognitive-Behavior Therapy for Late-Life Insomnia. *Journal of Consulting & Clinical Psychology,* 61:1, 137–46.
2. Froggatt, W. (2003). *Choose to be Happy: Your step-by-step guide.* Auckland: HarperCollins.

Chapter 13

1. Robb, Harold B. (1992). Why You Don't Have a 'Perfect Right' to Anything. *Journal of Rational-Emotive & Cognitive-Behavior Therapy*, 10:4, 259–270.

Chapter 14

1. Schultz, Duane P. & Schultz, Sydney E. (1990). *Psychology and Industry Today*. New York: MacMillan.

Chapter 15

1. Lakien, Alan. (1973). *How To Get Control of Your Time and Your Life*. New York: Signet.
2. The 80/20 rule — also known as the 'Pareto Principle' — was developed by economist Vilfredo Pareto.
3. For further guidance, see: Aslett, Don. (1984). *Clutter's Last Stand*. Cincinnati, Ohio: Writer's Digest Books.
4. Froggatt, W. (2003). *FearLess: Your guide to overcoming anxiety*. Auckland: HarperCollins.
5. For material on 'time-extension', see: Levinson, Jay Conrad. (1990). *The 90-Minute Hour*. New York: Penguin.
6. For more guidance on dealing with procrastination, see: Ellis, Albert and Knaus, William J. (1977). *Overcoming Procrastination*. New York: Signet.
7. See: Frank, Milo. (1989). *How to Run a Successful Meeting in Half the Time*. New York: Simon and Schuster.
8. Schlenger, Sunny & Roesch, Roberta. (1989). *How to be Organized in Spite of Yourself*. New York: Signet.

Chapter 16

1. Cash, Grady. (1994). *Conquer the Seven Deadly Money Mistakes*. 11225 Russian River Court, Rancho Cordova, CA: Center for Financial Well-Being (http://www.ns.net/cash/).

Chapter 17

1. Asimov, Isaac. (1978). My Own View, in Holdstock, Robert (ed). *The Encyclopedia of Science Fiction*. London: Octopus Books.

2. Toffler, Alvin. (1970). *Future Shock*. London: Pan Books.
3. Holmes, T.H. & Rahe, R.H. (1967). The Social Readjustment Rating Scale. *Journal of Psychosomatic Research*, Vol. 11, p. 213.
4. Toffler, Alvin. (1990). *Powershift: Knowledge, wealth, and violence at the edge of the 21st century*. New York: Bantam Books.
5. Sheehy, Gail. (1996). *New Passages: Mapping your life across time*. London: HarperCollins.
6. Imber-Black, Evan and Roberts, Janine. (1992). *Rituals for our Times*. New York: Harper Perennial.
7. Huxley, A. (1959). *Collected Essays*. New York: Harper.

Chapter 19

1. Froggatt, W. (2003). *Choose to be Happy: Your step-by-step guide*. Auckland: HarperCollins.
2. A 'creditor's pool' consists of a list of one's creditors. All creditors are contacted and their agreement obtained to be paid off over a period of time. Weekly or monthly payments are made to each creditor from the money available to the pool for that period, each creditor's share depending on how much they are owed.

Chapter 20

1. Bramson, Robert M. (1990). *Coping with the Fast Track Blues*. New York: Doubleday.
2. Loftus, Mary. (1995). Frisky Business: Love at work. *Psychology Today*, 28:2, 34–85; Mar/Apr.
3. Colbert, Audrey. (1989). *Dealing with Sexual Harassment: A New Zealand handbook for employers/employees, students and educators*. Wellington: GP Books.
4. Schmidt, Stuart M. & Kipnis, David. (1987). The Perils of Persistence. *Psychology Today* (Nov): 32–34.
5. Zuker, Elaina. (1991). *The Seven Secrets of Influence*. New York: McGraw-Hill.

6. Ellis, Albert. (1972). *Executive Leadership: A rational approach*. New York: Institute for Rational Living.
7. Bartol, Kathryn M. & Martin, David C. (1991). *Management*. New York: McGraw-Hill.
8. Summers, L.S. (1983). Stress Management in Business Organizations. *The Industrial-Organizational Psychologist*, 20:3, 29–33.
9. Sartain, A.Q. & Baker, A.W. (1978). *The Supervisor and the Job*. New York: McGraw-Hill.

Chapter 21

1. Palmer, Stephen & Szymanska, Kasia. (1994). A Checklist for Clients Interested in Receiving Counselling, Psychotherapy or Hypnosis. *The Rational Emotive Behaviour Therapist*, 2:1, 28–31.
2. Seligman, Martin E.P. (1994). *What You Can Change and What You Can't: The complete guide to successful self-improvement*. Sydney: Random House.

Index